Gestational Trophoblastic Neoplasia

A Guide for Women Dealing with Tumors
of the Placenta, such as Choriocarcinoma,
Molar Pregnancy and Other Forms of GTN

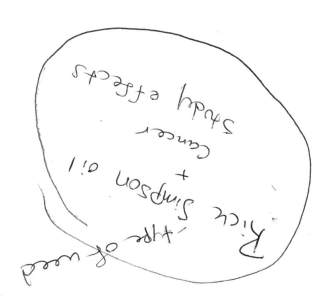

Gestational Trophoblastic Neoplasia

A Guide for Women Dealing with Tumors of the Placenta, such as Choriocarcinoma, Molar Pregnancy and Other Forms of GTN

Tara Johnson & Meredith Schwartz Ph.D.

*Foreword by Susan C. Modesitt, M.D.,
Associate Professor, Gynecologic Oncology Division,
University of Virginia*

Gestational Trophoblastic Neoplasia: A Guide For Patients Dealing with
Tumors Of The Placenta such As Choriocarcinoma and Other Forms Of GTN
Your Health Press
Copyright© Tara Johnson, Meredith Schwartz and Your Health Press, 2012.

Important Notice:
The purpose of this book is to educate. It is sold with the understanding that the
author and publisher shall have neither liability nor responsibility for any injury
caused or alleged to be caused directly or indirectly by the information contained
in this book. While every effort has been made to ensure its accuracy, the book's
contents should not be construed as medical advice. Each person's health needs are
unique. To obtain recommendations appropriate to your particular situation, please
consult a qualified health care provider.

All trademarked products appear herein minus the registered trademark symbol.

Design of print and digital editions: Anita Janik-Jones
Cover photo: istockphoto.com

ISBN: 978-0-9859724-4-8

ACKNOWLEDGEMENTS

We'd like to thank Susan C. Modesitt, M.D. and Wendy Hansen, M.D., whose expertise helped to ensure the accuracy of the information in this book. Ned Schwartz donated his time and artistic abilities to provide us with the images we required. M. Sara Rosenthal, Ph.D. gave us encouragement and guidance throughout the book's writing. Larissa Kostoff spent many hours tightening the structure and prose of early drafts, for which we're very grateful. We'd also like to thank Duane Hill for providing us with some of the articles that we used as source material.

We're indebted to Juliana's mom, Sarah Conyers, Sarah Dupuis, Heather Jackson, Candace Latourelle, Janet Lawrence, Angi Marek, Joanna Pugsley, Jacquie Radin, Vida Basilisa Roman-Boey and Georgette Roenelt for sharing their stories with us.

Tara would like to thank her husband, TJ—the love of her life—for always being there for her.

Meredith would like to thank Ms. Marion Clarke, whose dedication as a teacher instilled in her a love of the written word. She'd also like to thank her parents, Mary Ann and Paul Schwartz, who nurtured her desire to write, and her partner, Joel Swedburg, for giving her the time and support required to finish this book.

TABLE OF CONTENTS

FOREWORD

Susan C. Modesitt, M.D., Associate Professor, Gynecologic Oncology Division, University of Virginia

Meredith Schwartz and Tara Johnson have compiled a remarkably thorough book designed for women facing gestational trophoblastic neoplasia (GTN). The diagnosis of GTN is a very confusing and frightening event for women facing potentially serious complications from either an abnormal pregnancy or, rarely, a normal pregnancy. The authors combine the personal experiences of Tara, who suffered from choriocarcinoma following the birth of her daughter, with a comprehensive look at the types of GTN, the causes, and the treatments that are available. This will be a useful resource—both for women facing GTN and healthcare practitioners who may not be familiar with this disease process, as so little lay literature is available on this topic.

INTRODUCTION

When I found out that I was pregnant, my husband TJ and I scheduled our first visit with an OBGYN. That visit, and those that followed, convinced us that all was well. It was a "normal" pregnancy that culminated in the birth of my daughter, Tatum. I was ecstatic. Although I had a stepson, she was my first child. You could say I was willingly "born" into motherhood—and loving it.

Then things started to go wrong. I became tired all the time. No big deal, I thought, I had a newborn to look after: of course I was tired. I experienced the usual six weeks of postpartum bleeding—and then some. I was told (and had read) that this happens sometimes, and that I shouldn't worry about it. So, I didn't. I thought: that's what you get after not having a period for nine months. I bled off and on, with cramps to go with it. Sometimes the cramps were just annoying and other times they were really painful.

Before finally being diagnosed, I was admitted into emergency for hemorrhaging. The doctors did blood tests, and told me I had been pregnant again, and had probably miscarried. They kept me overnight and did an ultrasound, which came up clear with no fetus. The OBGYN let me go home the next day, informing me that it was either a miscarriage I experienced, or that a part of the placenta from the birth of my daughter had been left behind, and my body was trying to get rid of it. She gave me her card and told me that if I was still bleeding in two weeks I should call her office to make an appointment.

Two weeks later I was still bleeding. I called the doctor's office and was told that I couldn't get an appointment for a month and a half—and this was after I explained my situation to the receptionist. A month and a half later I was still bleeding. Finally I got in to see the doctor. She checked to see how much I was bleeding and told me to come back in two weeks if nothing had changed. After those two weeks passed I was again told that the next available appointment was in a month and a half. Of course I kept the appointment, and this time the doctor scheduled a D&C (dilation and cutterage) in yet another two weeks. *All this waiting!* It took a total of four months to get proper treatment! The doctor also gave me a prescription for the painful cramps I'd been having—to treat an infection "down there."

I got the D&C done and was called back for bloodwork the next day. I could tell something was wrong. The doctor told me that an "abnormal amount of tissue" had been found. She repeated herself, emphasizing the words "*a lot.*" She told me that she'd requested the bloodwork to ensure she'd gotten all of the tissue. She had not. The next day the receptionist called to ask that I come in again. No problem, I said. Then she told me to make sure to bring my husband. My heart jumped. I thought: *this is really bad.*

I was diagnosed with choriocarcinoma on February 7, 2002, when my daughter was almost nine months old. I was devastated to hear the words "you have cancer of the placenta." I sat there with this stupid grin on my face, holding back the tears. What a dreadful thing to hear—the words still ring in my ears to this day. I mean, *cancer!* Sure I had heard of it—lots—but I didn't know anyone personally who had had it before. All I knew about cancer was that it killed many, many people each year. Yet there I was, faced with it, being lead blindfolded into it by a gynecologist who didn't seem to know much more than I did. She said she'd never had a patient with this type of cancer before, and then she set up the necessary tests. My husband TJ and I went home.

TJ had to work that night, so I invited my friends Meredith and Danielle over for moral support. Meredith came armed with *The Gynecological Sourcebook* by Dr. M. Sara Rosenthal, which had a section on gynecological cancers. In it was a list of questions to ask your doctor. Together Danielle, Meredith and I tried to make the best of the situation, as well as learn something about this type of cancer. We laughed, we cried and, when we weren't glued to the television to take our mind off things, we focused on cancer.

The next day I phoned my doctor's office and explained that I had some questions. I got an appointment that afternoon. I think I scared my doctor with these questions and how prepared I was, because she got really nervous and began to blame the cancer on the doctor who'd delivered Tatum. We never will know exactly what caused the cancer, but I do know now that it could have been caught a lot sooner. My OBGYN even admitted being mad at herself for not catching the cancer sooner, and asked me how that could have happened. I told her about the four-month wait before the D&C, and she didn't even apologize. This really made me mad because I felt I had entrusted her with my life. I know that we all make mistakes, but this was not something I felt could be shrugged off.

And yet that's exactly what had happened.

Once diagnosed, my first treatment was scheduled for February 14, 2002.

Since I was diagnosed so late, the tumor had grown and spread through my uterine wall. As the chemo started to shrink the cancer cells, a hole in my uterus quietly and surreptitiously developed. On the morning of February 15th I was crippled by abdominal pain. I told my nurse how uncomfortable I was and how much pain I was in, and she brought me a Tylenol. I couldn't keep it down, and ended up vomiting it into the tub she'd provided. I told her I felt like I was in labor, and she brought me a Tylenol-3. After that, I vomited on the floor. I only vaguely remember being told by the head nurse that they were taking me down for an ultrasound. I needed to have a bowel movement and I felt like I couldn't move to go to the bathroom. Blood came out into the basin. The nurses thought one of my ovaries had erupted, and so they wheeled me down to get that ultrasound. I had to wait to get in.

I was almost unconscious from the pain and the loss of blood. I could barely breathe and my body was shaking so badly I was getting really annoyed. It seemed to take forever to do the ultrasound and the pressure on my abdomen made it hurt even more. The doctor asked me if it was alright to do an internal ultrasound. I nodded, yes. The doctor and the radiologist talked while examining me but I couldn't hear them, or focus on what they were saying. The internal ultrasound hurt even more. A couple of nurses in the room were trying to take blood from me, but my veins had collapsed.

After finding out exactly what was wrong (I was bleeding internally from my uterus), the nurses quickly wheeled me into the emergency and told the ER nurses to prep me for surgery. I remember hearing one of them suggesting that they leave me by the wall, and my doctor being very firm with her, and strictly saying "No. Prep her *now*—she's lost over four liters of blood." There were probably 10 people prepping me for my emergency hysterectomy. They put a catheter into my bladder, and IVs into the main artery in my neck and pelvis area. I couldn't feel them. All I was thinking was, "I hope this is over soon."

I barely managed to whisper to a nurse that my husband, TJ, was up in my room. I asked this nurse to go and get TJ; he had no idea what was going on. I had called him at work before going down for the ultrasound to tell him that I was in pain, and that I couldn't talk. And he'd come to the hospital thinking that one of my ovaries had burst.

All I could think now was that I had to be freed from the pain, the shakes and the terror of not being able to breathe.

When I got into the OR a nurse asked me to take off my gown. Another nurse looked at the first and said "yeah, right"—and then he cut the gown off for me. I was put under.

My parents and my mother-in-law flew from Saskatchewan to Toronto that day. Turns out I scared everyone, including myself, and yet it took me a while to realize that I'd almost died. At which point I also came to realize (and deal with) the fact that my husband and I wouldn't be able to have any more children together. However, I recovered from the hysterectomy quite quickly. Surgical techniques have improved and my scarring is minimal compared to what it would have been had I had the operation ten years ago.

This was my introduction to the cancer experience. I had a very severe case, although some women have experienced worse. Chances are that your case will be less severe than mine and you may experience fewer complications than I did.

What I hope is that this book will prevent a similar saga from happening to you. By reading about and understanding gestational trophoblastic neoplasia (GTN), you'll know when to press for earlier appointments or more information. Although my friend Meredith and I had heard of cancer (who hasn't?) neither of us had heard of GTN or choriocarcinoma before the diagnosis. Choriocarcinoma is rare form of GTN: it occurs in just 1 out of every 40,000 pregnancies. We began to search out information on choriocarcinoma and other gestational trophoblastic neoplasias (GTNs). As it turned out, this was not an easy task. Because GTN and choriocarcinoma are so rare, there is very little information available. We discovered that libraries had no books on the subject, so we turned to the Internet. There we found that different websites had different, or contradictory, information. One site would describe choriocarcinoma as "extremely curable," and the next (to our horror) would say that it was nearly always fatal. Obviously, information on the Internet is not always credible. But with no published material to use as a guide, we struggled to sort the "reliable" from the "unreliable" when it came to information about choriocarcinoma. We asked my doctor for advice, and he confirmed that there was nothing written on the subject aimed at the lay reader. He seemed reluctant to elaborate, and answered subsequent questions with the words: "Why do you want to know that?"

Meredith and I realized that we'd have to find out about this disease on our own. We began to look through medical journals. There, we found enough information to begin to get a picture of this group of placental disorders. We read and we wrote down questions. We filled a filing cabinet with medical studies and statistics, sociological studies and notes. A friend, Duane, came from Saskatchewan with piles of information that he had found as well. Meredith and I decided that we should write down what we'd learned so that other people with a similar diagnosis would have an easier time becoming informed. Essentially, we decided to write this book to fill a gap in cancer information.

There is no such thing as a "good" cancer. Choriocarcinoma has both good and bad aspects. On the positive side, it's one of the most curable types of cancer. And even though it spreads rapidly, between 75 and 95 percent of women diagnosed with choriocarcinoma will go into remission. The medical prognosis is often quite good. On the negative side, however, it's also a very difficult cancer due to the circumstances under which it occurs. Choriocarcinoma is associated with a pregnancy. It can be the result of a molar pregnancy, a tubal pregnancy, a miscarriage, or even a normal pregnancy. In some of these situations, the woman and her partner are dealing with the loss of a pregnancy as well as the added stress of chemotherapy. On the other hand, after a term pregnancy, the family in question has been blessed with a new life and new responsibilities—an adjustment for any couple—only to be told that they also have to adjust to cancer. Because of circumstances like these, we wanted a book on choriocarcinoma to cover both the factual aspects of the cancer, its medical side, and the subjective aspects of the cancer, its emotional side. Naturally the two are linked, and as such we've also included a description of the rigors of treatment, that is, what it's like to live through a course of chemotherapy. We focus on choriocarcinoma, because that is what I experienced. We have also included some information on other forms of GTN. Chapter 2 is specific to choriocarcinoma, but all other chapters apply to any form of GTN.

Meredith and I are a unique team. I've become an expert on choriocarcinoma through my own experiences with its diagnosis and treatment, while Meredith (at the time of this writing) is a doctoral student in the field of bioethics, and has researched extensively on medical issues. We set out to write a book that would combine our skills, share our story *and* answer your questions.

When Meredith asked me to participate in the writing of this book, I was so excited. I knew it would be a lot of work, but I wanted to learn more about what was happening to me, as well as help out others who would go through this cancer after me. When we first started the work, I found it hard to go back to my diary, to read and "relive" all of the things I had been through. No doubt a lot of that had been pushed to the back of my mind, to deal with later on, since my mind and my body had a lot to deal with already. But in writing this I've realized that as hard as it was for me to go through the cancer experience, it was also unimaginably hard on my family and friends. They were forced to "watch" me go through it, knowing they could do little to help make it better. Even Meredith sometimes found it difficult for her to write this book. She tells me it was hard for her to think about the possibility that something further might happen to me.

We decided to use my voice as the narrator of the story, since this book is really about what happened to me. Any time you read something in the first person *(I or me)* you'll know it's me speaking. Whenever the book shifts to Meredith's point of view, you'll notice we've used her full name. You'll also notice that we've dedicated an entire section to Meredith's "experience" of my cancer. Otherwise the book is organized around the questions we had about GTN and choriocarcinoma. We begin with medical questions and information, and then move into the social and emotional side of a cancer diagnosis. But do feel free to read the book in any order you think is important to you.

The first four chapters answer general questions about gestational trophoblastic neoplasia (GTN). Chapter 1 addresses the basics of GTN, to give you a clearer idea of exactly what your doctor means by the words "you have GTN." We also list some statistics on GTN from around the world. In chapter 2 we look at the specifics of what causes cancer and choriocarcinoma. We begin with an overview of cancer and then discuss the specifics of choriocarcinoma. Chapter 3 deals with the signs and symptoms of GTN. And chapter 4 discusses diagnosis and staging of GTN, the tests that your doctor will recommend and what those tests will measure. This chapter also includes a section on how to choose and deal with your doctor. The next two chapters discuss available treatment options and their effects. Chapter 5 deals with the conventional medical treatments that may be recommended by your doctor, and what these treatments entail. Complementary and alternative therapies are outlined briefly here as well. Chapter 6 looks in detail at the side effects of treatment, as well as how best to deal with these side effects.

The last three chapters delve into the emotional and social side of a diagnosis. Chapter 7 explores the importance of personal relationships and intimacy, which can be a source of both strength and stress. Chapter 8 addresses some of our collective fears about GTN and its treatment by looking at the fears *we* had going in. We discuss some of the things that could go wrong during treatment, including loss of fertility, developing a resistance to the chemotherapy protocol, recurrence, and death. Finally, chapter 9 looks to the future, and what that future holds for a woman who has survived GTN. This chapter discusses issues like the possibility of pregnancy after GTN treatment and delayed emotional reaction to a diagnosis, and ends with some lessons we've been taught about life as a survivor.

The back of the book also contains some very useful information. The resource list will help you continue to educate yourself about GTN, as well as connect you to support communities near your home and online. And, since a diagnosis of GTN carries with it a whole new vocabulary, we have included a glossary at the back of the book to describe many of the medical terms that are likely to come up during the course of this treatment.

We hope that you enjoy reading this book and that you find the information in it helpful. The material presented here is intended as a guide. Some sections may make you uncomfortable. That's OK. Each person will cope with GTN, cancer or miscarriage in her own individual way. And remember, when diagnosed with such a rare disease, it's normal to feel alone. We hope this book helps you to realize that there are others out there who share your experience, and that resources *do* exist.

CHAPTER ONE

UNDERSTANDING GESTATIONAL TROPHOBLASTIC NEOPLASIA

GESTATIONAL TROPHOBLASTIC NEOPLASIAS

"Gestational trophoblastic neoplasia" is an accurate description. "Gestation" refers to pregnancy and highlights the fact that this group of conditions is the result of conception. "Trophoblast" is the medical term for the placenta and highlights that this is a group of disorders of the placenta. "Neo" means "new" and "plasia" means "growth." So when put together, the term "gestational trophoblastic neoplasia" describes a group of conditions that result from conception and that involve an abnormal and unrestricted growth of placental tissues. Until recently, gestational trophoblastic neoplasia was called "gestational trophoblastic disease." The new name, GTN, was adopted in 2000 because it's more informative. In this chapter we'll examine the various different forms of GTN and how they are related to one another.

Under the umbrella of GTN you'll find molar pregnancy, invasive mole, metastatic mole, gestational choriocarcinoma and placental site trophoblastic tumors (PSTT). The first two conditions are not cancerous, although they may be *pre-cancerous*. Choriocarcinoma and PSTT *are* cancers. All diseases included in this group are disorders that originate in the cells of the placenta. Most people have never heard of these disorders—unless of course they've gone to medical school, or have themselves been personally affected (or have a friend or family member who has been affected) by one of them. Although the umbrella term "GTN" applies to all of the placental disorders that we discuss, we will highlight when the information we present also pertains to PSTT because it has unique characteristics that require separate discussion. In general, if we have not specifically indicated that we are discussing PSTT, you should assume that the information provided does *not* pertain to PSTT. Here is what one of the women we interviewed said about discovering that she had GTN:

> "I felt I was in a blur. The terminology [was] all new to me. As I recall my first doctor said that I did not have cancer but [what I had] might lead to it if untreated. I could not connect what kind

of a disease is this that needs chemotherapy but is not cancer? I could not understand when she said on the one hand that I had nothing to worry about but in the next vein told me to go on leave for one year. *One year?* This doctor confused me." – (Diagnosed at 36 in 1993; treated in Manila, Philippines and Kuala Lumpur, Malaysia.)

The easiest way to explain what causes GTN is to start with an examination of the normal development of the embryo and placenta, before exploring just what can go wrong.

NORMAL DEVELOPMENT

During normal development of a baby a single egg, produced by the mother, is fertilized by a single sperm from the father.

Diagram 1.1: Sperm and Egg Fusing

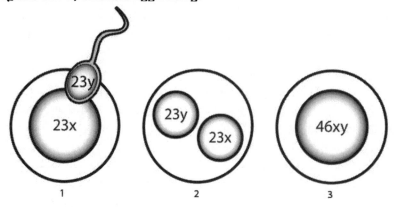

Egg cells and sperm cells are unique types of cells in the human body because each contains only 23 single chromosomes. All other cells in the body contain 23 pairs of chromosomes for a total of 46 chromosomes aligned in pairs. Again, egg and sperm cells have only half this number of chromosomes. However, the egg and sperm fuse in fertilization, thereby creating a complete set of 46 chromosomes. These chromosomes eventually align in 23 like pairs within the nucleus of the fertilized egg. The fused egg and sperm are then called a zygote. This zygote consists of a complete set of 23 pairs of chromosomes.

Diagram 1.2: First Stages of Development

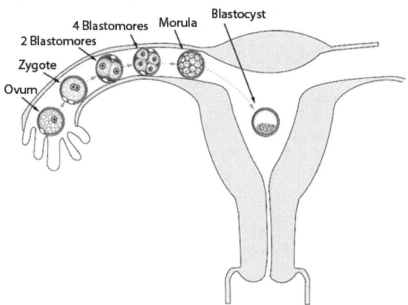

The zygote is the first stage in the development of a baby. The zygote is a single cell that derives half of its genetic information from the sperm of the father and half of its genetic information from the egg of the mother. The zygote has unique and complete genetic information. At this stage the developing baby is still in the fallopian tube of the mother. About 30 hours after conception, the zygote begins to divide. On the third day after fertilization, the embryo has 16 cells and has now entered the morula stage.

The morula is the name of the ball of cells that will become the baby and the placenta. At this stage the dividing cells are still using up the energy stores from the cytoplasm of the cells from the original zygote. No overall growth has occurred, although the number of cells has increased. The dividing cells are now becoming smaller than the cells that gave rise to them. An outer shell, called the zona pellucida, protects the ball of cells, or morula. The cells begin their journey towards the uterus at this point. This stage lasts for about four days, and then enters the blastocyst stage.

Diagram 1.3: First Stages of Development

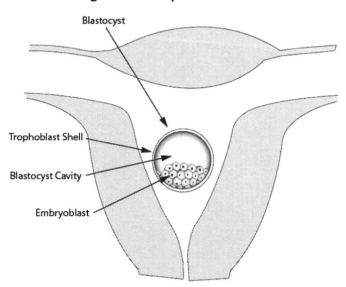

Blastocyst is the name of the stage of the developing baby at about day five, when the developing baby has reached the uterus. At this point the cells begin to segregate and form two distinctive parts: the inner layer of cells (called the embryoblast) will become the embryo and eventually the baby; and the outer-layer of cells (called the trophoblast) will become the placenta, the amniotic sac and the umbilical cord. The early blastocyst still benefits from the protective zona pellucida, but this outer shell will degenerate during this stage. After degeneration of the zona pellucida, the developing baby is called a late blastocyst. The degeneration or "dissolving" of the protective zona pellucida allows the developing cells to grow and expand. It also allows the embryo to obtain nutrients and oxygen from the uterine environment.

At about day six or seven of the blastocyst stage, implantation occurs, wherein the developing cells must attach themselves (implantation) to the lining of the uterus called the endometrium. This is important because the developing baby will soon require more nutrients and oxygen than is available without a blood supply. Implanting in the endometrium of the uterus via the placenta allows the baby to obtain the nutrients needed for growth.

The cells of the outer-layer of the blastocyst are composed of three parts that will eventually separate to become the placenta. These parts are: the syncytiotrophoblast cells, the cytotrophoblast cells and the intermediate trophoblast cells (collectively referred to as the trophoblast). The trophoblast cells produce human chorionic gonadotropin (hCG), and human placental lactogen (hPL). Human chorionic gonadotropin (hCG) is a hormone that allows the mother's body to continue to produce estrogen and progesterone, which will ensure that the lining of the uterus is maintained to protect and nurture the developing baby. Human placental lactogen (hPL) prepares the mother's breast tissue for milk production to feed the baby after birth.

Diagram 1.4: The Blastocyst

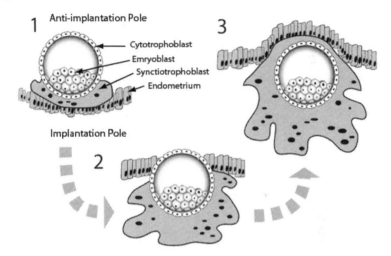

As the placenta grows, the syncytiotrophoblast cells release what are called "lysosomal enzymes" at the site where the blastocyst will attach to the endometrium. These enzymes create an "entrance" into the endometrium by eroding some of the tissue so that the blastocyst can penetrate into the nutritious tissue. As more synctiotrophoblast cells come into contact with the endometrium, the blastocyst is able to further penetrate into the uterus. Once the blastocyst is fully implanted into the endometrium, the erosion caused by the enzymes begins to heal.

After implantation the cells of the trophoblast begin to reproduce rapidly to produce microscopic finger-like structures that penetrate into the endometrium. These "fingers" are called chorionic villi (or villus to describe only one). The villi contain the fetal blood vessels needed to carry nutrients from the mother to the fetus. There are millions of villi in a placenta and each contains a single fetal blood vessel. The chorionic villi exchange nutrients, oxygen and metabolites with the mother's blood vessels without allowing any exchange of actual blood between mother and fetus.

Diagram 1.5: The Implanting Blastocyst

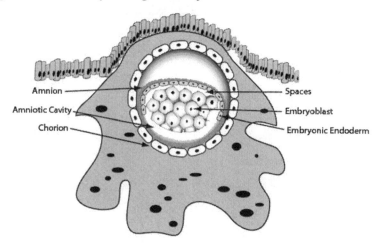

While the blastocyst is busy implanting into the endometrium, there are also changes occurring within the blastocyst. The cells begin to separate into the distinct parts that form the embryo, the amniotic sac and the placenta. The amnion and amniotic cavity eventually become the sac that protects the baby as it develops. This sac fills with fluid and is called the amniotic sac, which holds the embryoblast that will develop into the baby. The chorion becomes the chorionic sac, and this surrounds the amniotic sac. Between the seventh and twelfth weeks of gestation, the fetus has grown enough that the amniotic sac completely fills the chorionic sac, with the amnion pressing tightly against the chorion. This creates the single gestational sac present at delivery.

As development continues, the chorionic villi and the mother's blood vessels form a separate, distinct organ called the placenta. Normally, as a pregnancy progresses, the number of villi in the placenta initially increases— and then begins to decrease as the placenta ages. During the first week after

Diagram 1.6: The Developing Placenta

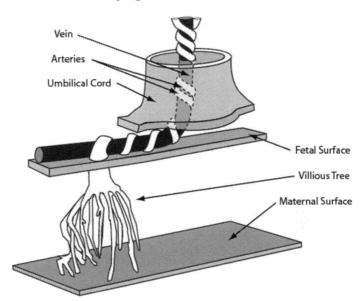

Vein

Arteries

Umbilical Cord

Fetal Surface

Villious Tree

Maternal Surface

implantation the inner mass of cells (the embryoblast) begins to differentiate and form the embryo, which will eventually develop into the baby.

The stage in the development of a baby during which the cells are dividing most rapidly is called the embryonic stage. In humans this stage occurs from about two weeks after fertilization until the end of the seventh or eighth week. Next is the fetal stage. It is during the fetal stage that the baby begins to take on a recognizable form. In humans the developing baby is called a fetus from about the end of the seventh or eight week until it is born.

After the birth of the baby, the placenta separates from the uterus. The doctor or midwife who delivers your baby should thoroughly examine the placenta (see pages 33–34) before it's discarded (or if you wish, kept for ceremonial purposes). This is to ensure that parts of the placenta have not been left in the uterus. You may also wish to take advantage of new technologies that allow parents to store cord blood, which is the same as infant's blood. This is carried out at the expense of the parents, and may be useful down the road in the event that the child requires stem cells.

DEVELOPMENT OF GTN AND CHORIOCARCINOMA

Sometimes things do go wrong during pregnancy. There are several problems that can occur, but we'll focus here only on those that give rise to gestational trophoblastic neoplasia. This group of problems or conditions consists of molar pregnancies, invasive moles, choriocarcinoma and PSTT. We will examine each in turn.

TYPES OF GTN

Complete Mole Partial Mole	Non-Cancerous
Invasive Mole Persistent Mole	Pre-cancerous
Metastatic Mole Choriocarcinoma Placental Site Trophoblastic Tumor (PSTT)	Cancerous

Molar Pregnancies and Hydatidiform Moles

Normally the combination of maternal and paternal genes is equal. This is important because it balances a baby's development. In all cases of molar pregnancy the relationship between the mother's genes and the father's is unbalanced.

Molar pregnancies occur when a fetus never develops but the placenta develops abnormally—and then continues to grow in an uncontrolled manner. This abnormal growth involves swelling of the villi and an overgrowth of the cytotrophoblast and synctiotrophoblast cells, causing the placenta to be abnormally large. The villi fill with water and grow in clusters that look like bunches of grapes. The placental cells produce a larger than normal quantity of hCG. Exaggerated symptoms of pregnancy can occur (including more morning sickness) along with vaginal bleeding from the abnormal placenta.

There are two types of hydatidiform moles, complete moles and partial moles.

Complete Moles

Complete moles contain no fetal tissue and are made entirely of placental cells. Complete moles occur when an egg that contains no genetic information is fertilized by one or more of the father's sperm. Sometimes when the egg cells are being formed in the mother's ovaries, the genetic information is not properly divided and one of the egg cells is without any chromosomes. If the egg is fertilized, the result is not a fetus, but a complete mole. Complete moles are called "androgenomic." 'Andro' refers to the male, and 'genomic' refers to the genetic information. The name simply describes the fact that in complete moles, all of the chromosomes come from the father's sperm, and there is no maternal genetic information.

Mole Fertilized by One Sperm

There are two ways a complete mole may arise. The first occurs when a single sperm with 23 chromosomes fertilizes an empty ovum (egg). These 23 chromosomes duplicate themselves to create 46 identical chromosomes. This is different from a normal situation in which a fertilized egg has 46 chromosomes, but the chromosomes pairs are not identical. In a normal fertilized egg, one set of chromosomes comes from the mother and the other set comes from the father. In this first type of complete mole, all of the chromosomes come from the single sperm. The result is a pregnancy with no fetal tissue; only placental tissue is present.

Diagram 1.7: The Complete Androgenomic Mole Fertilized by One Sperm

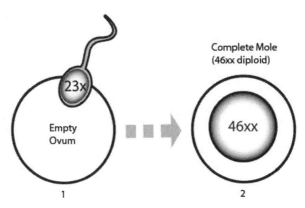

Complete Mole
(46xx diploid)

23x

Empty
Ovum

46xx

1   2

27

Mole Fertilized by Two Sperm

A complete mole can also occur when an empty ovum is fertilized by two sperms with 23 chromosomes each (called polyspermy fertilization). The fertilized egg has different chromosomal pairs, but all of the pairs contain the father's genetic information only. This genetic pattern also contains no fetal tissue; only placental tissue is present.

Diagram 1.8: The Complete Androgenomic Mole Fertilized by Two Sperm

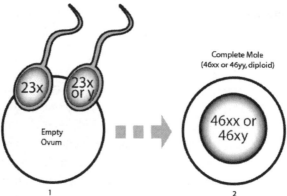

Partial Moles

A partial mole occurs when a normal egg from the mother (containing 23 chromosomes) is fertilized by two sperm from the father (containing, in each case, 23 chromosomes). This gives rise to a partial mole that contains 69 chromosomes (also known as triploidy). Partial moles usually contain some fetal tissue. But if a fetus is present it is most often abnormal with multiple malformations, as triploidy is incompatible with life.

When conception results in either a complete mole or a partial mole, "nature" often recognizes the genetic mistake. This will lead to vaginal bleeding and eventually a miscarriage (see pages 93–95 for more information). Most often the abnormal molar pregnancy is diagnosed by ultraound and then treated with surgery. Moles are initially treated with a surgical procedure called a dilation and curettage (D&C), sometimes referred to as a suction curettage (see pages 92–93 for more on these procedures).

Diagram 1.9: The Partial Mole

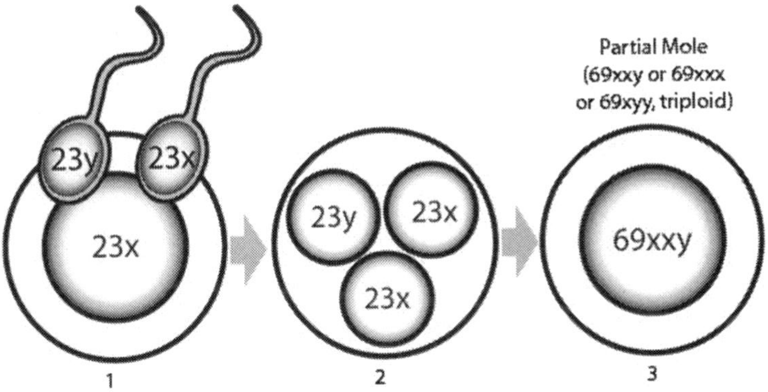

Partial Mole
(69xxy or 69xxx
or 69xyy, triploid)

23y   23x

23x

23y   23x

23x

69xxy

1   2   3

After removing the mole and uterine lining (endometrium), doctors will monitor your blood to make sure that treatment was successful. It is important that they look at levels of beta-hCG (a sub-type of human chorionic gonadotropin) in your bloodstream. This is because the beta-hCG of a woman with molar pregnancy may often be much higher (often in the millions) than it is in normal pregnancies. Measuring the amount of beta-hCG in your blood will let your doctors know if the D&C successfully removed all of the mole and placental tissue. Your blood will be tested every week until it's considered normal. Normal ranges are less than five.

Moles are not cancer, though they are sometimes treated with chemotherapy, especially when the initial surgery doesn't remove the entire mole or the mole already involved the uterine wall (see pages 85–89 for more on treating moles). Molar pregnancies are not usually a problem. Only about 20 percent of patients with moles will require chemotherapy after the initial surgery to evacuate the uterus. Usually, blood tests are normal within eight weeks. The cure rate for moles is nearly 100 percent

Following a molar pregnancy, your doctor will continue to monitor you with weekly HCG blood tests until they are normal. Once they are normal, your HCG levels will be tested monthly for at least 6 to 12 months. Problems can occur when molar pregnancies are ignored, or inadequately treated and followed. It's important to go to each and every one of your doctor's appointments to ensure that no problems have arisen. Your doctor will probably instruct you not to attempt another pregnancy for the year following a molar pregnancy. A normal pregnancy is not dangerous, but it will elevate the beta-hCG in the blood. This makes it impossible for your physician to determine—at least initially—if there is persistent disease present or just a pregnancy. During follow-up after molar pregnancy doctors look for several things: persistent moles, invasive moles, metastatic moles, or choriocarcinoma.

Persistent GTN or Persistent Moles

This category of GTN refers to moles *not* cured by dilation and curettage (D&C). Invasive moles may cause persistent GTN because a D&C removes only the inner endometrial layer of the uterus—and invasive moles may penetrate deep into the wall of the uterus. Most doctors prefer to use suction curettage because it removes more of the uterine tissue (see pages 92–93 for more information on these procedures). So do consider asking your doctor about this option. The survival rate for persistent GTN is nearly 100 percent.

Invasive Moles

Also referred to as chorioadenoma destruens, these are moles that penetrate the muscular wall of the uterus (called the myometrium). If a mole penetrates through the full thickness of the uterine wall it can cause a hole in the uterus, which may bleed heavily. Invasive moles are said to be "in situ" because they're located *only* in the uterus, and haven't spread anywhere else. Invasive moles are almost always caused by complete molar pregnancies, but rarely can occur after a partial molar pregnancy. Sometimes these moles disappear by themselves, but most require chemotherapy. This is because they've penetrated deep into the uterus, and may not be completely removed by D&C alone. Although a hysterectomy will eliminate the risk of local invasion after complete mole, hysterectomy can't prevent the mole from spreading to other areas, which happens in about 4 percent of cases of invasive mole. The survival rate for invasive mole is nearly 100 percent.

Metastatic Moles

In about 4 percent of cases involving a complete mole, and about 15 to 20 percent of cases involving an invasive mole, the mole may spread through the bloodstream to other areas in the body. If the mole spreads, it is called a metastatic mole. *Metastatic* simply means having the ability to invade other areas of the body. Invasive or persistent moles usually cause metastatic moles. The molar tissue in these cases has managed to leave the uterus (through the blood or lymph system) and has spread to other parts of a woman's body. Despite this, the survival rate remains excellent, and is about 97 to 100 percent.

Choriocarcinoma

This term is used to refer to one of the most aggressive and malignant (cancerous) form of gestational trophoblastic neoplasia. Worse, it's a form of cancer that can rapidly spread to other parts of the body. Cancer simply means that normal body cells have begun to grow out of control (see chapter 2 for a more detailed description of cancer).

The term choriocarcinoma comes from a combination of two words: "chorion," which is a Latin term that means "placenta" and "carcinoma," which refers to the type of cancer that it describes. "Carcinoma" refers to tumors that develop in the cells that line various tissues. Carcinomas make up 80 to 90 percent of all human cancers. "Sarcoma" is the other type of cancer. It refers to cancerous cells made up of connective tissue and accounts for only 2 percent of all human cancers. If the cancer is "in situ," it's confined to one place. If it's "invasive" (or metastatic), it has spread to surrounding tissue, lymph nodes or other organs.

Choriocarcinoma can develop from a molar pregnancy, an ectopic (tubal) pregnancy, the miscarriage of a healthy fetus, the therapeutic abortion of a normal fetus or, in rare instances, after a term pregnancy. If the preceding pregnancy was molar, your doctor should monitor you to watch for the development of choriocarcinoma. If the pregnancy was normal, then nobody would expect choriocarcinoma to develop. Choriocarcinoma is often missed after a normal pregnancy, and this oversight can give it time to spread dangerously before it's caught.

Choriocarcinoma is a very aggressive cancer because of the invasive nature of the placental cells that give rise to choriocarcinoma. Remember when we described the normal implantation of the chorionic villi into the endometrium? (If not, review the section that discusses "Normal Placental Development" on pages 22–25.) It's this feature of the placental cells that allows them to be so invasive. Even the normal invasion of these cells into the lining of the uterus is similar to the invasion of a cancer. It's natural in a healthy pregnancy

31

to find some placental cells throughout the mother's body; placental cells are very good at spreading. Normally, the cells are meant to invade maternal tissues and initiate the growth of new blood vessels, but the invasion is balanced by other genes that slow placental growth. In the case of choriocarcinoma, however, the invasion goes unchecked.

The good news is that the placental cells that give rise to choriocarcinoma are also very responsive to chemotherapy. Because the invasive action of the placenta is meant to be short-lived and responsive to "balancing" signals that slow placental growth, choriocarcinoma cells are primed to respond to chemotherapy. The treatment of choriocarcinoma usually results in a complete remission and seldom involves recurrences. The survival rate for choriocarcinoma is 75 to 100 percent, depending upon the risk group.

Placental Site Trophoblastic Tumor (PSTT)

This cancer is characterized by tumors found in the place where the placenta was attached to the uterus and in the muscle of the uterus. PSTT is another cancerous form of GTN. Like all forms of GTN, PSTT tumors are made of placental cells. However, other forms of GTN are composed of different types of placental cells than PSTT, which is composed mostly of syncytiotrophoblast cells. Unlike other trophoblastic cells, these cells do not produce hCG, thus the levels of hCG are lower for this type of tumor than they are for other forms of GTN. Measuring the hCG level is not as useful for determining the tumor load. Instead, the doctor will use an ultrasound or MRI to measure the extent of the disease. PSTT cells do not usually spread to other sites in the body, although they do sometimes penetrate through the wall of the uterus. Most patients with PSTT are treated with a hysterectomy since this tumor does not respond well to chemotherapy. About 50 percent of placental site trophoblastic tumors occur after a term pregnancy. This form of GTN is more likely than other forms to recur, so careful follow-up monitoring is essential. The survival rate for PSTT varies greatly (between 20 and 100 percent) depending on how many years elapsed before it was detected. Much of what is written in this book will not apply to PSTT since it has very different characteristics and treatment than the other forms of GTN.

RISK FACTORS FOR GTN

A risk factor is anything that increases a person's chance of getting a disease such as cancer. The baseline risk for a molar pregnancy in the United States is about 1 in 1,000-1,500 pregnancies. Choriocarcinoma occurs in approximately 1 in 20,000-40,000 pregnancies. Risk factors for GTN include:

- *Age.* The risk of molar pregnancy is higher for women who become pregnant over the age of 40, or before they have turned 20.
- *Prior molar pregnancy.* Once a woman has had a molar pregnancy her chance of having another ranges from 1 in 40 to 1 in 200. The risk is slightly higher than for a woman who never had a molar pregnancy.
- *Blood type.* Women whose blood type is B or AB are at a slightly higher risk than women whose blood type is A or O. This risk factor is controversial, and some doctors think that it should not factor into risk assessments.
- *Diet.* Some researchers think that women who don't get enough carotene or vitamin A in their diet may be at a higher risk for GTN.
- *"First Mating."* Some studies have suggested that the first pregnancy with a new partner provides a greater risk than subsequent pregnancies with the same partner.

Can GTN Be Prevented?

The only way to avoid the rare chance of developing GTN is to never become pregnant. There are no tests to determine whether one might be genetically predisposed to GTN. And there are no lifestyle factors that seem to be strongly associated with the development of GTN. So, in short, there is no way to prevent GTN, other than to avoid becoming pregnant. However, GTNs are so rare that no one would see the risk they may pose as a reason to remain child free. Studies have shown that women who've had choriocarcinoma are not any more likely to develop it a second time. However, women with a prior molar pregnancy are ten times more likely to have another molar pregnancy. Your chances of getting choriocarcinoma remain as low a woman with no history of this disease. (See pages 209–211 for more on pregnancy after GTN.)

Although it isn't possible to prevent choriocarcinoma, this type of cancer is much less serious if caught early. For this reason it's a good idea for pregnant women to ask about their hospital's placental triage policy. It's essential to have the placenta thoroughly checked for any abnormalities, such as damaged or absent ends (called cotyledons), which could signal that some placental tissue has been left behind in the uterus. This should be done after delivery of the baby. (For a good description of placental triage, see DSM PathWorks "Placental Triage 101," which can be found at: *http://showcase. netins.net/web/placenta/.)*

Please pass on this advice to any pregnant women you know. The inspection of a placenta is a gross—as opposed to a microscopic—observation, and thus cannot detect everything. However, the placenta *can* tell a lot about the health of the mother and the baby when it's examined by an experienced health professional. This examination shouldn't take more than a couple of minutes, nor should it ever be "shrugged off" by the doctor delivering. Knowing your rights as a patient is important, and it's the doctor's job to do his or her best in any situation of care. A doctor who doesn't take the time you need, or doesn't have an interest in answering your questions, listening to your symptoms or explaining something that you find hard to understand is not the doctor you deserve. For more on patient rights and dealing with your doctor, see chapter 4.

The Statistics for GTN and Choriocarninoma

- In Asian and African countries, GTN affects up to 1 in 2,500 pregnancies (American Cancer Society), although the reasons for the disease's higher incidence in this region are not known.
- Molar pregnancy affects approximately 1 in 120 pregnancies in Asia. In Northern Europe the incidence of molar pregnancy is 1 in 2,000 pregnancies. In the United States molar pregnancy occurs in 1 of every 1,500 pregnancies. (William Rich, 1996.)
- In very rare cases (approximately 1 percent) a molar pregnancy may occur along with a normal fetus. An example of this is in the case of fraternal twins, where one twin is healthy and the other is a hydatidiform mole (American Cancer Society).
- In approximately 10 to 17 percent of cases, a hydatidiform mole can progress to become an invasive mole or persistent GTN (American Cancer Society).

- Choriocarcinoma affects approxomately 1 in ever 20,000 to 40,000 pregnancies in the United States (American Cancer Society).
- 1 to 3 percent of hydatidiform moles develop metastatic GTN (American Cancer Society).
- 50 percent of choriocarcinomas develop in women following a molar pregnancy.
- 25 percent of choriocarcinomas develop in women following a spontaneous abortion, therapeutic abortion or tubal pregnancy (American Cancer Society).
- 25 percent of choriocarcinomas occur following a normal term pregnancy and delivery (American Cancer Society).
- Gestational trophoblastic tumors, taken together, account for less than 1 percent of female reproductive system cancers (American Cancer Society).
- All forms of GTN can be treated and, in the great majority of cases, treatment results in a complete cure. Nearly 100 percent of women with GTN who do not have complications can be cured.

CHAPTER 2

AN IN-DEPTH LOOK AT CANCER AND CHORIOCARCINOMA

CANCER BASICS

Reactions to a cancer diagnosis really vary. Many of us are shocked to learn that we've developed cancer. This is especially true of a cancer like choriocarcinoma, which tends to affect women who are young and still in their childbearing years. Here is what some choriocarcinoma survivors had to say about learning of their choriocarcinoma diagnosis:

> "To be honest I figured it might have been cancer or something just as serious, and my first thoughts were: *I'm going to die and I'm too young* and then *I got cancer from getting pregnant. How could this happen?*" (Diagnosed at 33 in 2002; Treated in Melbourne, Australia.)

> "I didn't find out about the cancer diagnosis right away. I had to pry it out of the doctors in the hospital, who kept calling it my "illness." I finally got a doctor to say the word cancer when I told him I'd refuse to do any more tests until I knew what was going on. I said: *Do I have cancer?* He said: *Do you really want to know?* I said: *Yes!* Back in 1973 doctors didn't like to tell patients they had cancer. They felt it was better to keep it quiet, to treat the patient and keep her as comfortable as possible until her demise. Even families weren't always told that a family member had cancer." (Diagnosed at 27 in 1973; Treated in Southampton, NY, and New York City, NY.)

If you feel unprepared at the beginning of your diagnosis, know that you're not alone. The next part of this book aims to paint a clearer picture of just what goes on in the body to produce cancerous cells. This will help you understand your diagnosis and make informed decisions about your cancer treatment.

A General Overview of Cancer

Cancer is an abnormal "mistake" in normal cell functioning. All cells in the body divide and reproduce in a cycle that's called the "cell cycle." This process is important to the body because in the young it allows growth, and in the old it allows the body to replace dying cells and repair damage to the cells that make up the body's systems. Once a cell has divided and replaced itself, the old cell dies. When a cell is functioning normally this occurs in an orderly fashion. Cancer occurs when some cells in a part of the body begin to grow out of control. The cells don't die when they're supposed to; instead they continue to live and continue to divide, creating more abnormally growing cells. But the cancer needs nutrients, which are carried in the blood. So the cancer begins to invade arteries to assure itself a steady supply of blood. It is this feature that gives cancer its name. Cancer means "crab" and refers to the crab-leg-like extensions formed by the blood vessels that supply blood to the cancer cells.

Cancer cells grow out of control because of damage that occurs to the DNA or because of "mistakes" during cell division. DNA is present in all cells. It regulates cell function and the production of proteins. Usually when DNA is damaged the body can repair it, but in cancer cells the damage to the DNA cannot be repaired. Damage to DNA can be inherited, as is the case with cancers that run in families. Other times the damage to the DNA is caused by the environment, as is the case with cancers that result from smoking or exposure to radiation. In still other cases, the damage is caused by a random "mistake" or malfunction in the way a cell is copied.

Because cancer cells are formed from cells that are already a part of the body, the immune system doesn't recognize cancer cells as problematic. The immune system thinks these cells are just like any healthy cell, and thus doesn't attempt to fight off the growth. This is why during the early stages of some types of cancer there are few symptoms. A tumor is simply a collection of many cancerous cells in a single area. The presence of the tumor causes problems due to the diverting of nutrients away from the healthy organ, which impairs the function of the normal body systems. Because the immune system doesn't recognize cancer cells as a problem, medical interventions are needed to destroy these cells.

Cancer cells often break off from the original tumor and spread through the blood stream or the lymphatic system to other bodily organs. This process

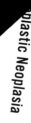
n the cancer cells reach these other organs they begin
: normal tissues. When cancer cells are growing on
air the functioning of that organ, and divert its blood
cancer you have is named for the organ it came from,
which it spreads. If you have choriocarcinoma with
metastases to ...., you still have choriocarcinoma, not lung cancer.

Different cells from different organs behave differently. Because cancer is made up of cells from these different organs, different cancers also behave differently. Choriocarcinoma is very different than breast cancer in growth rate, ability to spread and response to treatment. This is why people with different types of cancer receive different treatments.

Treatment will be aimed at the type of cancer you have. When the cancer cells have been killed as a result of treatment, and are no longer growing, you'll be in what's considered "remission." However, sometimes even after remission has been achieved a cancer begins to grow again. This is called a recurrence. If after five years you're still in remission and cancer-free, you're considered cured (although some types of cancer can still recur after five years).

This section provides an overview of the basics of cancer. Since this section is complex it isn't essential to read it until you feel you're ready. However, I've found it useful to have a grasp on the biological changes that occur in cancer because it gives me a better understanding of what exactly is happening in my body. Just picturing the cancer, or developing a mental image of it, also helps if you decide to try alternative therapies (see chapter 5 for information on complementary and alternative therapies). Many techniques use mental imagery to "break down" the cancer in your body, and in fact studies show that using mental imagery from the beginning of a diagnosis helps more than if this technique is adopted later on.

THE GENETICS OF CANCER

It takes many steps to turn normal, healthy cells into cancerous cells, a change that's called carcinogenesis. In this brief introduction to cancer genetics, we'll look first at the normal life of a cell (to help you understand what's *supposed* to happen), and then at the two most important genes that normally act to prevent cancer—proto-oncogenes and tumor suppressor genes. If you want a more detailed description of the genetics of cancer, a good article is: June Peters et al. "Cancer Genetics Fundamentals." *Cancer Nursing vol. 24 no. 6, 2001.*

The Cell Cycle and Normal Cell Function

Normally cell reproduction is an ordered and tightly controlled process. The cell cycle is a series of steps in which the start of a new step requires the completion of the previous step in a continuous loop. For a cell to divide and become two cells, several steps are necessary. The genome (DNA) must first be copied, the cell's mass must double in preparation for splitting in two, then the chromosomes and other cell parts must be segregated so that the two daughter cells have exactly the same make-up as the cell they came from. These events are divided into phases: first is synthesis (S), and then there is a gap or resting phase (G2). After this rest comes the phase called mitosis (M), during which chromosomes and other cell matter (mitochondria, ribosomes, cytoplasm, etc.) are evenly split into the two daughter cells. Finally there is another gap (G1) before the sequence begins all over again.

Diagram 2.1: The Cell Cycle

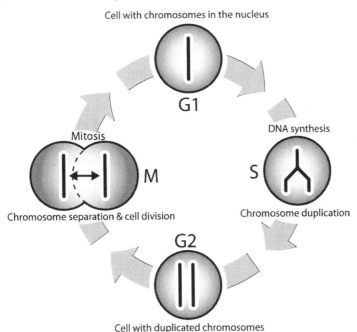

You may want to put a bookmark or sticky tab on this page so that you can refer to this diagram as you read about the cell cycle.

Sometimes after the second gap (G1), the cell goes into a resting phase (known as G0). If there's irreparable damage to the DNA, which is detected during the G0 phase, then the cell will sacrifice itself to help maintain the proper working of the rest of the organism. This process is called apoptosis.

The copying of DNA, chromosomes and their segregation only occurs during the synthesis and mitosis phases. Cell growth occurs continuously throughout the cell cycle. It is typically the G1 and G2 phase, when the cells are responding to the growth and antigrowth signals, that determines whether the cell will be copied or will come to a stop either temporarily (G0) or permanently. During the G1 and G2 phase there are cell cycle checkpoints wherein enzymes detect and repair any damage to the genetic material. If the damage is irreparable, the cell self-destructs (apoptosis). Events that disrupt or damage the cell's internal regulation system, trapping it in unending cycles of growth, are key events in the development of cancer.

Diagram 2.2: The Cell Cycle with Apoptosis

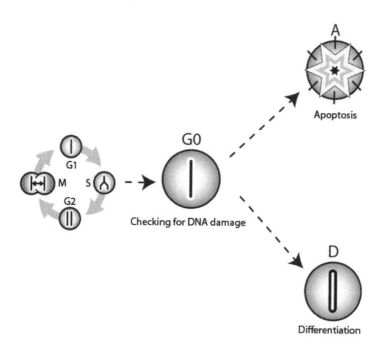

40

The Cancerous Cell

Let's now look at the two major players in the genetic development of cancer. These are the oncogenes and the tumor suppressor genes. Normally they function to prevent cancer, but sometimes they lose their ability to protect the cell from becoming cancerous. This is the first step for a cell on the road to becoming cancer.

Proto-oncogenes and Oncogenes

The normal cell process of growth, development and death is controlled in an orderly fashion by our genes. When genes are working well they're called proto-oncogenes. Proto-oncogenes make proteins that stimulate cell division and keep the cell alive (they inhibit apoptosis). We need proto-oncogenes to ensure that our bodies can repair the cellular damage that may occur from daily activity. That is why we can't simply "cut out" proto-oncogenes to avoid cancer—we need them!

In cancer development, mutations or other genetic alterations cause proto-oncogenes to start to produce their own signals. Instead of listening to the normal signals coming from outside the cell, they tell the cell to reproduce. The cell thinks it's receiving a growth message even when it isn't. Thus cells keep dividing and growing without end. If these mutations occur, the proto-oncogenes are now considered oncogenes.

A simple analogy may help clarify the function of oncogenes. Oncogenes are like a car's accelerator. If the car is working well, the accelerator allows the driver to go faster or slower depending on outside conditions and also the driver's pressure on the pedal. The mutations that give rise to cancer are like a mechanical problem that causes the accelerator to get stuck in the "down" position, creating a runaway car. It doesn't matter what the driver sees outside the window—it could be a stoplight or a police car—the driver can no longer decrease the pressure on the accelerator, so the car keeps going. The oncogenes cause the cell to keep copying itself out of control. When a cell begins to accelerate its growth out of control, the cell has taken the first step on the road to becoming a cancerous cell.

Tumor Suppressor Genes

Just as a car has more than one system to control its speed, cells also have more than one growth regulation system. A car has an accelerator, but it also has brakes. Tumor suppressor genes act as the brakes. Tumor suppressor genes are present in all normally functioning cells and are there to slow cell growth. In cancerous cells, these genes are missing or have become "broken" by mutations. This signals the loss of the cell's ability to slow its growth, and once again leads to unrestrained cell division.

Brakes are important to both cars and cells. In fact, because they're so important there are two braking systems in a car: the front and the rear brakes. Similarly there are two copies of tumor suppressor genes (called alleles), which can be likened to the two sets of brakes in a car. Just as having one functioning set of brakes is enough to slow a car, the cell only needs one copy of the tumor suppressor gene for slowing the growth of new cells. However, if both the first and second copies of the genes are lost, the cell is left without any working brakes. Tumor suppressor mutations are known as "loss of function" mutations, because, as long as just one set is working, they continue to slow growth. It's only once both copies have lost their function that cells become cancerous.

There are two types of tumor suppressor genes: gatekeepers and caretakers. Gatekeepers are those genes that produce proteins to directly regulate growth by stopping cell division or by promoting cell death (apoptosis). The inactivation of gatekeeper genes leads to unrestrained growth directly because the damaged cancerous cells are let through the gate.

Caretaker genes produce proteins that maintain the stability of the genome. The inactivation of caretaker genes contributes to tumor growth by causing an increased mutation rate. The increased mutation rate creates a greater chance that mistakes will happen that will give the cell cancerous characteristics.

Some genes, such as p53, can be both gatekeepers and caretakers. The gene p53 is thought to be very important in protecting cells from becoming cancerous. This gene is known as the "guardian of the genome" because of its role in detecting DNA damage. Either it repairs the damage or, if the damage can't be repaired, p53 sends the cell permanently out of the cell division cycle to its death. Some authors feel that p53 is an essential gene in carcinogenesis. Once the cell has lost its ability to slow its growth, it has taken the second step on the road to becoming cancer.

Specific Genetic Alterations in Choriocarcinoma

We've seen that there are a number of different steps that lead to cancer, and that the body has many places where it normally regulates and suppresses tumor growth. There are specific types of genetic alterations that take place in cancer development, but only some of these are relevant to choriocarcinoma. We'll examine the relevant changes in the next section.

THE GENETICS OF CHORIOCARCINOMA

Choriocarcinoma is a unique type of cancer. In all other cancers, cells from the patient's own body invade healthy tissues. Choriocarcinoma is different. In this cancer, cells from the embryo invade the mother's tissues. In other words, the tissues are invaded by cells that are actually genetically distinct from the mother.

Like all cancers the development of choriocarcinoma is a multi-step process and involves multiple genetic changes, including the activation of oncogenes and the inactivation of tumor suppressor genes. We end off the section on the genetics of cancer by mentioning specific genetic changes that occur in choriocarcinogenesis. Now we'll explore the genetics of choriocarcinoma.

Genomic Imprinting in Choriocarcinoma

As you now know, placental growth is normally balanced by maternal and paternal genes (see pages 24–26). This balancing occurs through a process called imprinting. Genomic imprinting refers to the fact that for certain traits, genes are chemically coded to show whether they come from the mother or the father. Genomic imprinting doesn't change DNA. What the gene controls will be different, however, depending on whether it comes from the mother or the father. Genomic imprinting is essential for the proper development of certain human features. For example, imprinting is thought to play an essential role in the development of the placenta. It has been suggested that maternal and paternal imprinted contributions to the embryo's genes are meant to balance the development of the placenta. *Paternally* imprinted genes stimulate the placenta to grow and invade the maternal endometrium, whereas *maternally* imprinted genes are meant to stop this from going too far. Maternal genes are meant to inhibit placental invasion. When this balance is disrupted, placental growth goes unchecked.

Imprinting explains why complete moles are more likely to turn into chorio-carcinoma: they lack any maternal genetic information and thus only carry paternal genetic information. Partial moles, where two sperm fertilize the same egg, are also explained by imprinting. In the case of partial moles, there is an excess of paternally imprinted messages and the placenta grows wildly. Partial moles are less likely to become choriocarcinoma than complete moles because they do contain some maternally imprinted genes to slow placental growth. It's unclear what happens in the rare cases wherein choriocarcinoma develops after a normal, healthy pregnancy. It may occur when placental cells lose their imprinting, and either the signals from the maternally imprinted genes are turned down, or the signals from the paternally imprinted genes are turned up.

Loss of imprinting is thought to be reversible. Researchers are looking into ways of restoring imprinting that may, in the future, give rise to new forms of treatment for choriocarcinoma.

The Role of Oncogenes and Tumor Suppressor Genes in Choriocarcinoma

We discussed the role of oncogenes and tumor suppressor genes on pages 41–42. Approximately ten different oncogenes and tumor suppressor genes are thought to be involved in the development of choriocarcinoma. The tumor suppressor gene p53 is mentioned at more than one checkpoint as a factor in the progression from non-cancerous placental tissue to choriocarcinoma. The purpose of the tumor suppressor gene is to repair DNA damage, so its presence may signal that the cell is trying desperately to repair itself by making more p53.

Placental Cells Achieve Immortality

Cells "live" by dividing in half and creating two identical copies of the original cell. Normal cells have a limited life span. They can only undergo a predetermined number of divisions before they are too old and "die." Within each cell there is a mechanism (called telomeres) that counts down the number of divisions the cell has undergone. This mechanism ensures that cells do not "live" past their expiration date.

The "countdown" mechanism is always on in adult humans, but it also has an "off switch." It's important that this mechanism has an "off switch," because we all begin as a single cell. During embryonic development our cells are dividing rapidly, and they are definitely not counting the divisions. If our cells *were* counting the divisions during embryonic development, we might run out of living cells before even being born! The "off switch" is called "telomerase," and is very important for proper embryonic development. In healthy adult cells there is no telomerase, and thus every cell division is counted.

In cancerous cells, the "off switch" somehow gets flipped. Cancerous cells stop counting the number of divisions that they're undergoing. Because countdown is "off," cancer cells can reproduce indefinitely. In a sense this scenario means that cancer cells have found the fountain of youth, and can therefore live forever. This is one reason cancer is difficult to cure. The cancer cells have extended their natural life span; they don't die on their own and thus must be destroyed instead by some outside agent (such as chemotherapy).

Studies have found that telomerase is present in choriocarcinoma cells. If there is telomerase in the cells of a hydatidiform mole, this increases the chance that the mole will proceed to become persistent trophoblastic disease, or choriocarcinoma.

Developing New Blood Vessels (Angiogenesis) and Invasion (Metastasis) in Choriocarcinoma

Cancer grows quickly and thus needs a constant supply of blood to carry nutrients to cancer cells. In order to ensure adequate nutrition, a cancer can actually cause the growth of new blood vessels in order to feed itself. This diverts the blood away from healthy organs and impairs the body's ability to function properly. And it is this feature of cancer, called angiogenesis, which gives the disease its name—since the new blood vessels leading to the tumor look like the legs of a crab.

It's easy for placental cells to stimulate the growth of capillaries and to invade tissues, because this is what these cells do even when they're healthy (see the section on normal placental development, pages 24–25). With a slight disruption (such as polyspermy fertilization, a mutation or loss of imprinting) of the genes that normally hold these processes in balance, the placental cells are able to spread. If other genetic changes have occurred to make the placental cells cancerous, then choriocarcinoma is the result.

CHAPTER 3

THE SIGNS AND SYMPTOMS OF GTN

IDENTIFYING THE SIGNS AND SYMPTOMS OF GTN

Signs and symptoms are an indication that there may be disease, illness or injury affecting the way a body is meant to function. This chapter will look at some of the signs and symptoms associated with GTN. However, it's important to remember that everyone's symptoms, diagnosis and personal experiences with GTN are different. Blaming your symptoms on other things (e.g., having a newborn or adjusting to the news of a miscarriage) is normal. But do make sure to tell your doctor about what you're experiencing and how you're feeling *at all times* so that he or she can treat you properly, and give you (or direct you to) the additional help you need. The lesson here?—you don't have to "tough it out."

Scattered throughout this chapter are the stories and experiences of women who have survived choriocarcinoma. Meredith and I met many of these women at a "yahoo"choriocarcinoma support group (see the resource list at the back for addresses and contact information). This group is for women who are experiencing life as chorio patients, and for survivors of chorio—who have chosen to help current patients by guiding them through their treatment. This group has really helped me get questions answered. Also, since choriocarcinoma is such a rare diagnosis, it's hard to find other women with whom to identify. Because the group is web-based, it brings together women from all over the world to create an insightful, helpful community of choriocarcinoma survivors.

What's the Difference Between a Sign and a Symptom?

Signs and symptoms are indications that something isn't right in the body. Signs and symptoms may be caused by a disease, illness or injury that is affecting one or many of the body's systems. Symptoms are subjective and are felt or noticed by the patient, but are not easily observed by anyone else. Symptoms are usually difficult to measure. Fatigue, weakness, aching muscles, shortness of breath and chills are all examples of symptoms. Signs are objective (e.g., vaginal bleeding, low blood count, etc.) in that they are easily observed or potentially measured by someone else, such as a doctor, nurse or other healthcare practitioner. Fever, rapid breathing, and rash are all examples of signs.

The presence of one sign or symptom may not be enough for a physician to figure out what is wrong. For example, a fever is associated with many different ailments. It's the combination of signs and symptoms together that give a physician the clues necessary to make a diagnosis.

Often a patient's signs and symptoms are not enough to tell with certainty what is wrong. A physician will have to call for other medical tests to be absolutely sure of making the right diagnosis. The combination of signs and symptoms gives your doctor a clue as to which diagnostic tests he or she should order (see chapter 4 for more on this). Some signs and symptoms are very noticeable. Others are difficult to detect, since a patient may just attribute them to the common discomforts of life. Here's what some of the women we spoke with told us about the way their choriocarcinoma symptoms affected their daily life:

> "Suffice it to say, this happened, and my life stopped, I was running my own business so that stopped also." (Diagnosed at 31 in 1994; treated in Cleveland, OH.)

> "I carried on with whatever I was doing. I was studying then and I'm a person with a one-track mind. As a matter of fact when I'm busy with something I forget most other things. I can even shut out hunger." (Diagnosed at 30 in 1997; Treated in Sheffield, UK.)

> "My first sign was that I collapsed, lost bowel control and bodily control on my right side. I was told I was pregnant and had gestational migraines. The symptoms did affect my daily life as I was at home with my daughter and suddenly needed 24/7 care in case I collapsed. I needed people to take of [my daughter] and myself, and to be there to watch [my daughter]. When I collapsed I ended up with a horrific migraine [that lasted] for a long time." (Diagnosed at 33 in 2002; treated in Melbourne, Australia.)

SIGNS AND SYMPTOMS SPECIFIC TO GTN

There are signs and symptoms that are specific to GTN. However, if the disease spreads because it isn't detected early enough, each woman with metastases will have different symptoms according to the area to which the disease has spread. This section will explore the signs and symptoms specific to gestational trophoblastic neoplasias, then we will look at general cancer symptoms that may indicate the presence of choriocarcinoma, and those signs and symptoms that are specific to different sites where the disease often metastasizes.

List of the Signs and Symptoms Associated with Gestational Trophoblastic Neoplasia

- vaginal bleeding
- anemia (meaning, low red blood cell count)
- abdominal swelling (especially if associated with molar pregnancy)
- pain (pain during intercourse and pain in the pelvic area)
- infection
- vomiting
- preeclampsia
- hyperthyroidism
- symptoms from other metastases

Vaginal Bleeding

This is the most commonly experienced sign of choriocarcinoma and GTN. Almost all women with hydatidiform moles will experience irregular bleeding during pregnancy. This bleeding usually starts in the first trimester between the 6th and 16th week of pregnancy. If you have a molar pregnancy you may notice blood clots or a watery brown discharge from your vagina. If the preceding pregnancy was normal there may or may not have been abnormal bleeding during pregnancy, but there will almost certainly be abnormal bleeding after delivery. If you notice that you're bleeding after you've delivered, have a doctor check for choriocarcinoma, especially if the bleeding persists beyond six weeks or is severe. If the tumor penetrates the uterine wall there can be bleeding into the abdominal cavity accompanied by severe abdominal pain.

After having Tatum, I didn't actually "stop" bleeding. It would be heavy for a few days then get light so it was like spotting. After a few days of bleeding ever so slightly it would get heavy again. Then, on the night of October 5th 2001, while we were having a birthday party for my stepson Tragean, I was confined to the washroom because I was bleeding so badly. I was passing clots the size of grapefruits. When I finally got a little break from the gush, I wore a towel to try to soak up the blood while my husband took me to the hospital emergency. Tatum was just over four months old. I was admitted to emergency right away and I was given blood tests. The doctor came in, asked how old Tatum was, and then told me that I had been about three months pregnant, but that I had probably miscarried. They did an ultrasound to see if I had a fetus in me. I didn't, so they assumed that I had already passed it. Little did they know the extent of their misdiagnosis.

Here is what some other women had to say about their experience of vaginal bleeding:

> "Light brown spotting for about six to eight weeks in first trimester and then heavy bleeding on the day of diagnosis" (Diagnosed at 30 in 1997; treated in Sheffield, UK.)

> "Three months after I delivered my son, I started to bleed. I thought my menstrual period was starting. But by afternoon, I was hemorrhaging profusely—there were clots the size of a large fist or larger. Whenever I stood up they just fell out of me. No pain or anything accompanied the hemorrhaging or clots. I called my doctor, who advised me to stay in a "reclining" position, and to make sure my feet were higher than my head. If the bleeding didn't stop by the next morning I was to call him and go straight to the hospital for a D&C. That's how they initially found the chorio." (Diagnosed at 27 in 1973; Treated in Southampton, NY and New York City, NY.)

Anemia

Anemia is a medical term for "low red blood cell count." If a woman is experiencing severe bleeding her body may not be able to replace all the red blood cells that are being lost. Symptoms of anemia are fatigue, shortness of breath and inability to exercise or engage in strenuous activity to the normal extent. About half of women who have gestational trophoblastic neoplasia will also have anemia.

Abdominal swelling

Molar pregnancies are associated with a larger uterus and, sometimes, larger ovaries. This makes the entire abdomen feel larger than what's considered the average for the same stage of pregnancy. The placenta is often more swollen than is usual, so the woman appears as though she could be six months pregnant when in fact she's still in her first trimester. About half of women with complete moles will experience this unusual swelling. It's more rare, however, in women with partial moles. Choriocarcinoma can also cause the uterus to expand. The hCG produced by the tumor may cause a type of ovarian cyst (called luteomas) that contribute to abdominal swelling.

Here is what one of the women we interviewed had to say about abdominal swelling:

> "...I was huge. I looked about five or six [months] pregnant and I was already in maternity clothes. The doctor thought I was having twins!" (Diagnosed at 30 in 1997; Treated in Sheffield, UK.)

Pain

Pain during intercourse and pain in the pelvic area are specific signs of GTN. After the birth of my daughter, I experienced pain in my pelvic area that felt like I was in labor again, but without the "break" in between contractions (although it would die down after a while). I also experienced pain during intercourse. I know that after having a baby intercourse is painful at first, but it didn't go away. It hurt everywhere—outside and inside. It felt as if my insides were all swollen, and most of the time we had to stop in the middle of having sex because it hurt so badly. Another symptom I had was an unusually dry vagina. I had to use a lot of lubrication before even starting anything intimate. (For more information on sex and intimacy please see chapter 7).

Here is what one of the women we interviewed said about the pain:

> "OHHHHH PAIN! Was I in pain! Horrible, horrible, pain. From the day I had my daughter I was in and out of the doctors' offices and hospitals. I had severe pains in my sides (due to the kidney and liver metastases) and severe pain in my left shoulder. I couldn't even move out of bed to use the restroom. I threw up anything that went into my body and not even pain medications were helping me. I couldn't stand up without passing out and I lived in my bed from the day she was buried to the day I was diagnosed. It

was actually a blessing to be diagnosed, because I knew that I was dying and if they didn't figure out was wrong to help me then I was going to die." (Diagnosed at 24 in 2001; treated in New York City, NY.)

Infection

The uterus may become infected due to the presence of GTN or choriocarcinoma. Infection in the uterus produces a vaginal discharge and crampy pain in the pelvis. I experienced pelvic cramps. The cramping was really more annoying than painful at first. But this developed into cramps that were as painful as labor pains. I would sit on the toilet hoping to "push something" out of my body. I didn't know what I was trying to push out; I only knew my body was telling me there was something wrong, and that I needed to get it out. At the same time, I was having a major bout of hot flashes and I had to strip down until I was naked. I would sit there on the toilet—naked, sweaty—and I'd have a tingly sensation throughout my body. This would last for 10 to 15 minutes and then would disappear, leaving me a little crampy for the rest of the day. It seemed to happen maybe once every two weeks at first, and then it became more frequent and more painful. I'd crawl from the toilet to our bed, crying and rocking myself in an attempt to deal with the pain. When I told my doctor, she prescribed some antibiotics because she thought I had an infection "down there." The cramps continued until my hysterectomy. I thought they were just menstrual cramps in the beginning, but it turned out they were a result of the choriocarcinoma.

Here is what one of the women we spoke with said about infection:

"I never in my life had a yeast infection until I was pregnant with my daughter. I had them almost the whole time I was pregnant with her. The doc just put me on medications for them." (Diagnosed at 24 in 2001; treated in New York City, NY.)

Vomiting

Vomiting is considered normal in pregnancy and is called "morning sickness." However, studies have reported that women with GTN experience more frequent and severe vomiting than is associated with a normal pregnancy. Some researchers think that the increased nausea may be due to elevated hCG levels. If you think that you're sicker than you should be, don't ignore it—and by all means don't just try to "be brave." Let your doctor know that you're feeling unwell and that you think it might be more than run-of-the-mill morning sickness.

Here is what some women we interviewed said about the vomiting:

> "I thought [I had] more than average "morning sickness" at the time but during the two pregnancies [I went through] after recovering from choriocarcinoma the sickness was the same… I was unable to go into work for much of the first three months of pregnancy due to sickness, bleeding, etc." (Diagnosed at 30 in 1997; treated in Sheffield, UK.)

> "When I was pregnant, I vomited so often that I didn't know what it was like not to vomit." (Diagnosed at 24 in 2001; Treated in New York City, NY.)

Preeclampsia

Preeclampsia is a medical condition characterized by high blood pressure, exaggerated reflexes and excessive blood protein in the urine. Preeclampsia is another condition that can be associated with a normal pregnancy or can be a sign of GTN. In a normal pregnancy preeclampsia usually occurs during the third trimester, but in molar pregnancy it often develops sooner, in the first or second trimester.

Hyperthyroidism

Hyperthyroidism occurs when the thyroid is overacting and is producing too much thyroid hormone. Hypothyroidism occurs in GTN patients due to the fact that hCG has a "subunit" that is virtually identical to the TSH (thyroid stimulating hormone) that stimulates the thyroid to produce more thyroid hormone. Symptoms of hyperthyroidism include rapid heartbeat, warm skin, tremors and feelings of being on edge. About seven percent of women with molar pregnancies also have hyperthyroidism.

After I had my hysterectomy, I had no idea what exactly had happened, and how it could affect my body. One of my friends had asked me how my thyroid would react to not having a uterus. So, I asked my first gynecological oncologist—let's call him Dr. "A"—if having a hysterectomy would affect my thyroid. He looked at me as if I was stupid, laughed, and said: "No—why would it affect your thyroid?" He then changed the subject, basically treating me like I didn't know what I was talking about. I really *didn't* know what I was talking about, and that's why I was asking *him!* Now that I know that elevated levels of hCG can cause the thyroid to become overactive, I am even angrier that Dr. A just dismissed my question, and treated me like a child. Not to mention the fact that one would expect a *gynecological* doctor to know about the effects of a hysterectomy on the thyroid. (For more information on hysterectomies, see chapter 5.)

Here is what one of the women we spoke with said about hyper-thyroidism:

> "I believe that I had this during pregnancy. Right before being diag-nosed with chorio I was in thyroid storm, but I believe I suffered from hyperthyroidism during pregnancy, and that was why I was losing weight while pregnant…and seeing the spots and passing out and feeling like my heart was gonna pop out of my chest." (Diagnosed at 24 in 2001; treated in New York City, NY)

Symptoms from Other Metastases

The symptoms that are caused by spreading will depend on where in the body the tumor spreads. If it spreads to the digestive system, there may be bloody stools or bloody vomiting. If the tumor spreads to the brain, there may be headaches, dizziness, seizures or paralysis on one side of the body. The next section will look at the general signs and symptoms associated with all cancers, plus some signs that indicate the cancer may have spread.

SIGNS AND SYMPTOMS THAT MAY INDICATE METASTATIC GTN

The rest of this chapter is specifically aimed at women who have metastatic GTN. However, if you have another non-metastatic form of GTN you may still want to read this section so that you will know what signs and symptoms to look out for that may indicate that your GTN has progressed further and become cancerous.

Cancer taken as a group of diseases together can cause virtually any sign or symptom. As cancer progresses it goes through many stages, and the signs and symptoms associated with these stages are different. The symptom produced will depend on the size of the cancer, the location of the cancer, and the surrounding organs or structures. Some signs and symptoms are common to all cancers; others are specific to the area that is affected by the cancer. If the cancer spreads (metastasizes), then the symptoms will also be different. The signs and symptoms will be specific to the kind of damage the cancer does in the organ to which it has spread. Again, these new symptoms will change as the cancer grows in its new location. If you're unlucky enough to experience metastatic cancer, you may also experience a variety of different symptoms as the cancer moves around your body.

As cancer grows it begins to exert pressure on the nearby organs, blood vessels and nerves. This pressure creates many of the signs and symptoms of cancer. If the tumor is in a critical area, such as the brain, then even a very small tumor may cause symptoms. If the cancer is in another location, such as the pancreas, there may not be any symptoms until the tumor has grown quite large, and has begun to exert pressure on the nerves. Cancer cells may release substances that alter the body's function. Cancer cells may also cause the immune system to react in ways that cause signs and symptoms of illness (e.g., fever).

It is difficult to specify signs and symptoms for cancer because every person's cancer has unique properties. It will have common symptoms if it originates in the same organ, but it will have unique symptoms if it spreads because each person's cancer may spread to a different location. Two women with choriocarcinoma will have some common symptoms (those associated with having a cancer growing in the uterus) but they'll also have unique symptoms if the cancer spreads to other areas in the body.

Despite the difficulty involved in pinpointing them, it's very important to recognize and pay attention to symptoms. Symptoms tell us that something is wrong in the body. The treatment of cancer is most successful when the cancer is caught early. Many patients miss or ignore symptoms because they don't recognize that the symptom itself is significant. Fatigue, one of the key symptoms of cancer, is often dismissed as "just part of life." But these symptoms should never be overlooked, especially if they last for a long period of time (such as several days or a few weeks).

Signs and Symptoms of Cancer

The *general* signs and symptoms of cancer are those common to most cancers. The *specific* signs and symptoms of cancer are those that represent a unique response to the cancerous tumor's location. Listening to your body is good for you. All symptoms have a cause, and all deserve to be checked out. The signs and symptoms discussed in the section below apply only to the malignant forms of GTN. Even if you've been diagnosed with a non-metastatic form of GTN, you should know what to watch out for so that you can alert your doctor to any possible signs that your GTN is progressing.

General Signs and Symptoms Common to All Cancers

If you have cancer you'll probably experience some or all of these signs and symptoms. It may help to keep a symptom journal so that you can see if there's a pattern to when you feel ill. This could point to some lifestyle factor or dietary event that may be aggravating the signs and symptoms of the cancer.

General Signs and Symptoms Common to All Cancers

- weight loss
- fatigue
- pain
- skin cues

Weight loss

Most people with cancer experience weight loss at some point in the course of their disease. Unexplained weight loss of about 10 pounds may be the first sign of cancer. This sign is especially significant for cancers that originate in or have spread to the pancreas, stomach, esophagus or lungs. In my case, detecting the weight loss was somewhat confusing, as I had a term pregnancy so it was normal for me to lose weight after delivery. However, I did lose those pregnancy pounds very quickly. I am a small person to begin with, so I thought it was just my body getting back to its regular size. A friend who had given birth a couple of days after me kept commenting on the amount of weight I had lost and how quickly I was losing it. It got to the point where I weighed less than my normal weight—10 pounds less, to be exact. I really didn't think anything of it at the time. I (along with everyone else) thought I was lucky that I didn't have to "work off" those extra pounds. I guess I wasn't so lucky after all!

Here is what one of the women we interviewed said about weight loss:

> "During my pregnancy I had weight loss. But after, I lost even more weight. I was about 30 pounds lighter when I was diagnosed

with cancer than I was before I got pregnant with my daughter."
(Diagnosed at 24 in 2001, treated in New York City, NY)

Fatigue

Fatigue is often a symptom of cancer as it progresses. Fatigue may occur early, especially if the cancer causes a loss of blood, as is often the case with chorio-carcinoma. But as we discussed earlier, blaming symptoms on things in your life is easy. I felt really drained and tired before being diagnosed—but I had a brand new baby to take care of! Who wouldn't be tired? However, I didn't lose that tiredness at all as my daughter got older. I just got more tired and more drained. I'm lucky that my baby was very good and had no problems with colic, as I probably wouldn't have had the energy to take care of her or the rest of my family.

Here is what some women we interviewed had to say about fatigue:

> "I had no energy and was tired all the time. But I thought that was just being pregnant that was doing that to me." (Diagnosed at 24 in 2001; treated in New York City, NY)

> "I began to feel drained a lot more often." (Diagnosed at 33 in 2002; treated in Melbourne, Australia)

Pain

Pain is often a symptom of advanced cancer. In many cases it is caused by the cancer growing so large that it begins to exert pressure on the nerves or other organs. I started to get unusual sharp pains in my ribs. It wasn't a constant pain, just hard stabbing pain that would come and go (this was from the cancer spreading to my lungs). I also had cramping pains that felt like I was in labor again (due to the presence of cancer in my uterus). I was crippled over and in tears.

Skin Cues

Some internal cancers can cause visible changes to the skin, such as redness (called erythema), itching, darkening of the skin and excessive hair growth. The only thing I experienced in terms of skin cues was an abnormally long-lasting linea nigra (the dark line that appears down the middle of the belly in the last six months of pregnancy). Like most women, I got the dark line from the navel to my pelvic area. Usually this line goes away within a couple of months after delivering. Mine has only recently disappeared, and it's nearly two years since I gave birth to my daughter.

Signs and Symptoms Specific to Different Areas the Cancer May Spread

The signs and symptoms discussed in the following section refer to specific locations to which the cancer may spread. These signs and symptoms apply only to metastatic GTN or other cancers. You'll only experience them if the cancer has spread to the location associated with these cues. If you do experience any of the signs and symptoms below, let your doctor know immediately. It may mean that the GTN has spread to a new location and is causing problems there.

The Most Common Sites for Metastases from GTN

Pay extra close attention to any signs associated with these locations!
- lungs (80 percent)
- vagina (30 percent)
- brain (10 percent)
- liver (10 percent)
- gastrointestinal (GI) track, kidneys and pelvis (20 percent)

Lung Symptoms

The lung is the most common site for distant metastasis of choriocarcinoma or other forms of metastatic GTN. If the cancer spreads to the lungs you may cough up bloody mucus. You may also experience a persistent dry cough, chest pain or trouble breathing. I experienced all of these symptoms. I had eight tumors growing on my lungs. The symptom that scared me most was coughing up blood. My first chemo treatment had me in the hospital overnight while they were administering the drugs. I had a major "dry coughing" attack and coughed up blood. The nurse put a humidifier on in the room and it hasn't happened again since. The other symptoms—chest pain, trouble breathing and persistent cough with and without mucus—occurred on a daily basis. Since I was a smoker, I blamed it on the smoking. However, the doctor told me that I hadn't smoked for long enough for that to be the cause. Rather, it was due to the cancer spreading to my lungs.

Here is what we heard about lung symptoms from one of the women we interviewed:

> "I would start out by having trouble breathing then see the spots then pass out. This was very scary. But I happened all the time, just either out of the blue or if I stood up too quickly, walked too much, anything would set it off." (Diagnosed at 24 in 2001; treated in New York City, NY.)

A nagging cough or hoarseness that doesn't go away are signs that there is cancer present in the lungs. Since this is a common site of metastases for choriocarcinoma these are signs to watch out for. Hoarseness can also be a sign that there is cancer in the voice box (larynx) or thyroid.

Vaginal Mass, Unusual Bleeding or Discharge

You may also notice abnormal growths on the vagina, labia or vulva. These growths may indicate that the tumor has spread to these locations and has begun to grow there.

In GTN, the persistent or invasive placental tissue in the uterus often bleeds significantly, so bleeding from the vagina may signal the presence of continued disease—and may not mean the cancer has spread to distant areas. However, blood in the urine can also signal that the cancer has spread to the kidneys or the bladder. If there is blood in your pee be sure to let your doctor know right away. After having Tatum I was "menstruating" off and on until I had my hysterectomy. It would get really heavy for a few days and then fizzle out to spotting. Then, it would get heavy again. I had no idea what was wrong, but it was really annoying. This went on for nine months. I also had the usual menstrual cramping to go along with it. This only became understandable after I found out it was due to the choriocarcinoma.

Brain

Often metastasis in the brain causes few symptoms until the tumor has grown so large it has begun to exert pressure on the brain. This may trigger headaches, dizziness fainting or collapsing. Headaches may signal that the disease has spread to the brain, but this can be tricky because sometimes the elevated hormone levels associated with GTN may also cause headaches. It's best to be safe and check with your doctor.

"[I had] headaches and I also had a stroke followed by two brain hemorrhages. Although I don't remember this time, I am told I was in great pain." (Diagnosed at 31 in 1994; treated in Cleveland, Ohio)

"I started having migraines. I had five in seven days. I hadn't had a migraine in over three years. My migraines I believe are linked with hormones." (Diagnosed at 32 in 2000; treated in Ontario, Canada.)

Changes in Bowel Habits or Bladder Function

Chronic constipation, diarrhea or a change in the size of the stool may indicate that cancer has spread to the colon. Pain when you pee, blood in the urine, or a change in how often you need to pee may signal that there is cancer in the bladder. It's important to watch for these signs since these are common sites for choriocarcinoma metastasis. These signs may be hard to detect because choriocarcinoma originates in the uterus, it can grow and exert pressure on the bladder and may cause changes in urination even if it hasn't spread to the bladder.

CHAPTER 4

DIAGNOSING GTN AND CHORIOCARCINOMA

Identifying GTN in the early stages isn't always possible. This is because the signs and symptoms of GTN are very much like those of a normal pregnancy. A doctor will often naturally assume that you're pregnant, and not affected by a disorder. Fortunately GTN is very treatable, even when it isn't detected until the later stages, after metastasis has occurred. When a doctor suspects that you may have GTN he or she will probably recommend that you undergo a series of tests to determine whether the disease is localized (in situ) or has spread (metastasized). After these tests the doctor will be able to determine the extent of the disease in your body. The doctor will then look at these results and assign a "stage" to the GTN. The staging system looks at risk factors and helps a doctor to determine a prognosis (a medical prediction of how difficult the cancer will be to treat and how aggressive the treatment needs to be).

This chapter takes a close look at these tests and the reasons a doctor will order them. Remember: *you may give or withhold your consent to each test.* If you're uncomfortable with any one of the tests for any reason you have the right to refuse to give your doctor permission to perform the test. This chapter will give you an idea of what the tests measure; that way you can weigh the benefits of the test (e.g, what information it provides) against the burden you feel the test might impose (e.g., how invasive it is, or what level of discomfort you'll be expected to tolerate). If you feel that the burdens outweigh the benefits, then you don't have to consent to the test.

I found that the actual tests the doctors perform aren't as bad as waiting for the test results to come back. My doctor put a rush on all the tests I went through, so I only had to wait a couple of weeks at the most. That's including the time in between scheduling, the tests themselves, and getting the results. I was advised of all the possibilities in terms of where the chorio could have spread. Just waiting to see how bad it actually was was very stressful. I had problems sleeping and concentrating and was extremely emotional (thinking that it had spread and that it wasn't going to be at all curable), even though my doctor was very positive about the outcome, whatever the results.

Here's what some of the women we interviewed had to say about their experience with taking these diagnostic tests and hearing their diagnosis:

> "From beginning to end I was diagnosed with kidney stones, kidney infections, bladder infections, depression and hyperthyroidism. The kidney stones and depression were misdiagnosed. I definitely had hyperthyroidism, and I'm not sure whether the infections were real or not. I took medications for them but the pain never went away, so I think they were misdiagnosed—and the pain was actually from the tumors in my kidneys and bladder. After all these tests were performed over a period of a month and a half, I wound up in the intensive care unit, and the docs still couldn't figure out what was wrong with me. Finally a gyno on call came in and asked me if he could call the hospital I delivered my daughter at, and have the pathology department re-check the placenta. That was when I was finally diagnosed with chorio. I felt great when I was diagnosed with cancer. I know that sounds weird, but I was just so glad that they finally knew what it was, and also that they could now start to make me feel better. I did not know the stage I was in until after I was almost better. They informed my husband that I would probably die, and explained to him how far the cancer had spread. They kept it a secret from me because they didn't want me to get even more upset, and not be able to keep my good spirits up. I'm actually glad they did this for me, because I know that I would not have been as strong as I was if I knew I was supposed to be dying." (Diagnosed at 24 in 2001; treated in New York City, NY.)

> "First of all I wasn't told at the time of the diagnosis what stage I was in. I didn't learn this until much later. I felt ill when I was told the diagnosis. I couldn't breathe. I thought I was in a bad dream. I was told I was two to three months pregnant four days before I was diagnosed. This was a misdiagnosis." (Diagnosed at 32 in 2000, treated in Ontario, Canada.)

THE TESTS FOR ALL FORMS OF GTNS

There are several tests that are performed to determine the extent of the disease and whether or not the disease has spread to other parts of the body. The tests fall into the categories of pelvic exam, imaging tests and blood tests.

Pelvic Exam

The pelvic exam that looks for GTN should be carried out just like any other physical that you've had in the past. The only difference is that instead of screening for *possible* problems, the doctor already suspects there is a problem, and will focus on the signs that might indicate GTN.

A doctor should perform this exam with the presence of a nurse chaperone. If desired, you can also request the presence of family or friends. Don't hesitate to ask for this service if you desire it. If your doctor makes you feel uncomfortable, however, that might be a signal to you that you should find a different doctor (we'll return to a discussion of how to choose your doctor at the end of this chapter). On the other hand, you may also ask any observers to leave if their presence is bothering you. Your doctor may request that you allow medical students to observe your case. While many patients enjoy the opportunity to contribute to the education of future doctors, you're not obliged to participate. The choice is up to you.

Speculum and Bi-manual Pelvic Exam

The manual exam tests for an enlarged or abnormally shaped uterus. The doctor will have you lie on the examination table, undressed from the waist down. The doctor will then use a speculum to open your vagina in order to see the walls of your vagina and your cervix. The doctor will look to see if there are any unusual growths on the vagina, labia and vulva. If there are growths, this may indicate that the disease has spread to the outer organs of the vagina. And if the doctor sees growths he or she will probably order more diagnostic tests to determine conclusively just what is causing them.

The doctor will also reach two fingers inside your vagina and place one hand on your belly, over your uterus. He or she will then apply a slight pressure to feel for any abnormal masses in the uterus, or to see if the uterus is an abnormal shape. This test is not perfect for detecting choriocarcinoma because the lumps formed by this type of cancer are often too small to be felt. Most gynecologic oncologists will then also perform a rectovaginal exam, wherein one finger (the index finger) is kept in the vagina and the middle finger of the same hand is placed into the anus/rectum. While this can be disconcerting and uncomfortable, it allows the physician to assess the posterior of the uterus and pelvis.

When I had my pelvic exam, I was very uncomfortable. The doctor who checked me out was okay, but the resident really hurt me. This procedure was weird for me because I didn't know what to expect, and I really don't think that it should have hurt at all. Needless to say, I switched doctors after the first one didn't listen to my request not to have the resident doctor looking after me in any capacity.

Pap Smear

During the speculum examination, your doctor may want to do a Pap smear. This tests for the presence of abnormal cells on the cervix; it is a screening test for cervical cancer and not a diagnostic test for spread of GTN. The Pap is done by gently scraping some cell samples from the cervix. The doctor uses a small brush to rub the cervix, which causes some cells to shed. The cells are then put in a preserving solution and sent to a lab for analysis. This test may indicate whether or not the disease has spread to the cervix. I found this test was much more comfortable for me than the bimanual exam (as comfortable as you can get when you're laying there half naked and someone is checking out your vagina!). It wasn't painful at all, and felt very routine. It lasts a couple of minutes (if that)—but then of course there's the waiting for results.

Biopsy

If your doctor suspects that you have choriocarcinoma he or she may order a biopsy depending on the circumstances. The word "biopsy" is derived from the Greek, and it loosely translates as "view of the living." Most cancers are confirmed by a biopsy. However, in the case of GTN the biopsy may cause extensive bleeding, so your doctor may think it best to avoid this risk. Because of the risk of bleeding, biopsies are most commonly ordered only for GTN patients who've had a D&C or hysterectomy. When a biopsy is performed, a small sample of the suspected cancerous tissue is removed from the patient and sent for pathological examination. The pathologist who examines the tissue is a specially trained physician who can determine the cause of symptoms by examining tissues or fluids from the patient. The pathologist performs a series of tests and then sends the results back to the patient's physician. When I had a biopsy done, my OBGYN sent tissue for examination after my D&C. This is how she found out about my choriocarcinoma.

Imaging Tests

Imaging tests are most useful for determining if your GTN has spread to other organs. The doctor uses these diagnostic tools to look at your abdomen, pelvis, chest and brain to check for the presence of tumors in these locations.

X-Rays

X-ray machines use waves of electromagnetic energy. These waves are directed through your body. A small window in the X-ray machine lets some of the X-rays escape in a narrow beam. The beam passes through a series of filters on its way to your body. The X-rays then create different patterns when they encounter different tissue types.

A camera on the other side of you records the pattern of X-ray light that passes all the way through your body. The X-ray camera uses the same film technology as an ordinary camera, but X-ray light sets off a chemical reaction instead of visible light. Harder areas of the body (such as bones and dense tissue masses, like tumors) appear whiter on the X-ray negative. The X-ray may miss smaller and softer tissue abnormalities, so a doctor will often order more imaging tests rather than relying on X-rays alone.

When I went in for the X-rays that were ordered on my lungs, the technician made me wear a hospital gown because I was wearing a shirt that had a picture on it. I was asked to take my bra off. Then the technician positioned me in front of a backdrop. I put on a heavy lead apron that snapped like a belt around my waist, and was told me to take a deep breath and hold it while the X-ray was being taken. The technician took two pictures, one from the back and one from the side.

Computer Assisted Tomography Scan (CT Scan or CAT Scan)

A CT scan is a special X-ray procedure involving a scanner, which rotates around the patient and directs variously angled beams of X-rays at a particular region of the body. The computer combines these images to produce a detailed cross-section of the body. Some CT scans require the use of a radioactive dye. If you have any allergies to shellfish and are undergoing a CT scan, you should let your doctor know, as sometimes the dyes that are used cause an allergic reaction in people with shellfish allergies.

I was quickly scheduled for an appointment to undergo a CT scan after I was diagnosed with chorio, to see whether or not I had brain metastasis. I had never had a CT scan before, and so I had no idea what to expect. After I walked in for my appointment, they immediately "prepped" me. I went into a separate room where I was given a hospital gown to change into. I then had to hop up onto a bed and answer the usual questions—to make sure I was the right person they were prepping! The nurse inserted an IV, and sent me to the waiting area. After a while, I was called in for the scan. The CT technicians made me take out all my earrings (because jewellery interferes with the picture they're able to get of the brain). I lay down on the bed as the technicians explained, briefly, what was about to happen. The technicians hooked up the dye to my IV and inserted it intravenously (although most people also have a certain amount of time to drink a liquid dye). This creates a tingly feeling in your bottom (like you have to pee, which they warn you about!) and it also caused a metallic taste in my mouth. The technicians went into the other room and proceeded to do the test. The bed moved into a circular "cove" that was somewhat closed-in, though not so much that I became claustrophobic. The laser spun around and around, and I could hear the humming of it. You aren't supposed to move throughout all of this, but they do tell you when it's *really* important not to move. It lasted maybe 5 to 10 minutes, and then it was over. It's just waiting for the results that sucks, even if you get them that day, or the day after!

A couple of the women we spoke with had several CT scans:

> "I had a lot of these. I had to swallow about three cups full of the dye, which I needed to do for the scan. And they wanted me to hold that in my bladder [which was] tough going. Sometimes they needed to inject a dye by IV too. Some patients are allergic to this dye, so if they suspect you are allergic they premedicate you prior to the scanning" (Diagnosed at 36 in 1993; treated in Manila, Philippines and Kuala Lumpur, Malaysia.)

> "The day I had the CT scan I was feeling extremely nauseous. My Beta-hCG was approximately 250,000 at this point, and I had to drink a liquid, which I could only barely get down after they put an IV in my arm with gravol. I took a vomit dish to my scan appointment." (Diagnosed at 32 in 2000; treated in Ontario, Canada.)

Ultrasound

Ultrasound uses sound waves like sonar. The pattern of echoes produced when the sound waves reflect off *normal* tissues is different than the pattern produced by a reflection off GTN cells. Some very slightly colored jelly is first rubbed on your abdomen (hopefully it's been sitting on the warmer, or else it's really cold!) The ultrasound technician uses a probe (called a transducer), which moves around on the jellied area on your body to get a picture of what's happening, or to see what's wrong inside of you. The transducer picks up the echo patterns that are translated by a computer into images, which can be viewed on a screen. The picture is called a sonogram. Most of the time, the technician won't tell you what he or she sees, unless you get a really nice one. This is because the technicians are not trained to read the results of the tests, and are worried about interpreting them incorrectly. You can often get technicians to "warm up" by asking questions, and letting them know that you realize they're not experts in interpretation.

If the ultrasound technician can't see, or would like to get a clearer view, you may be asked to do an internal ultrasound. In this case, foam padding is put beneath your tailbone and a probe is inserted into your vagina. The ultrasound technician then moves this probe around to get the pictures he or she needs. This isn't painful at all, but a little uncomfortable because you're lying upright with something inside you (unless you're bleeding internally, in which case any ultrasound is painful).

For any abdominal ultrasound procedure you need to have a full bladder (although you will need an empty bladder for an internal or vaginal ultrasound). The procedure takes about thirty minutes and can be somewhat uncomfortable because your bladder is full. You may have heard that you need to drink four to eight glasses of water per hour the morning of your ultrasound in order for your bladder to be full. Really this is too much for most women. One glass of water per hour should be fine. If you need to pee, then you've had enough water. If your bladder is *very* full before you leave for your appointment, call the clinic to find out how long you'll have to wait. If it's going to be a while, pee before you leave for your appointment. There's no sense sitting in a waiting room trying to keep from peeing only to wait another hour and a half (during which time you could have built up more for the test!). If you feel painfully uncomfortable while you're in the waiting room, go to the bathroom and only pee out half. And if you've misjudged and don't feel the urge to pee when your name is called, ask the receptionist to put someone ahead of you and drink some water while you wait for your turn.

Magnetic Resonance Imaging (MRI)

MRI scans use powerful magnets and radio waves to create a cross-sectional view of the body. MRI scans are more detailed than CT scans. The magnets are very powerful and the MRI should not be used by a patient with a pacemaker. Be sure and alert your doctor if you have a pacemaker. Some women find that the MRI makes them feel claustrophobic. If you have issues with claustrophobia, you can ask about the possibility of an "open" MRI (although these are new and are not available in all regions). You may also request special mirror-glasses to allow you to see a loved one standing at the open end of the MRI tube.

Many of the women we spoke with found the MRI to be a long procedure. Here is what they said:

> "The MRI scan I found very scary—being inside the machine and on my own—although not painful or uncomfortable." (Diagnosed at 30 in 1997; treated in Sheffield, UK.)

> "The blub-blub sound of the machine was irritating. I found the procedure too long for my comfort. In retrospect I guess at the time I had this test I was going through a lot of chemos and other testing, so my level of tolerance had grown thin." (Diagnosed at 36 in 1993; treated in Manila, Philippines and Kuala Lumpur, Malaysia.)

> "Yes [I had an MRI]... I hated the feeling of being closed in the tube." (Diagnosed at 41 in 2002; treated in Pensacola, Florida.)

Blood Tests

Blood tests measure the amounts of different substances in your blood. There are tests to measure the amount of placental cells, which is indicated by measuring a substance called beta-hCG for most forms of GTN (all forms of the disease other than PSTT). The amount of this substance in the blood has a direct correlation with the number and size of the placental growths in your body. Knowing how much placental growth you have allows your physician to plan your treatment properly.

Serum hCG

This blood test measures the amount of hCG (human chorionic gonado-tropin) present in the bloodstream. The test looks for hCG because this hormone is produced by placental cells, and therefore can indicate if placental cells are present in the body. This is the hormone that's detected by most pregnancy tests that you'd take at home or at the doctor's office. Usually the presence of hCG indicates that a woman is pregnant, because under normal circumstances the only time there are placental cells present in a woman's body is when she's pregnant. However, since GTN involves the placental cells that are growing *despite* the fact that there's no pregnancy, the presence of hCG can also signal the presence of choriocarcinoma or other forms of GTN. This marker is very accurate. In fact there's a direct correlation with the extent of the GTN and the amount of hCG found in your bloodstream. The higher the hCG count, the more extensive the disease in your body.

The normal beta hCG count varies slightly depending on what your hospital considers a normal range, usually between 0–4 and 0–5 for non-pregnant women. When I found out I had cancer, my count was 556,000. Having higher hCG levels doesn't necessarily mean that your GTN has spread; however, it likely means that the number of placental cells is larger.

The hCG levels can be detected in several ways. The women who had their hCG measured by drawing blood were more satisfied than were the women who had their hCG tested by a lumbar puncture (although this is very rare). Here is what they said:

> "This test was easy but painful on the pocket, as it was an expensive test in the Philippines. [I] am glad my treatments were followed up in Kuala Lumpur, where the tests were a whole lot cheaper." (Diagnosed at 36 in 1993; treated in Manila, Philippines and Kuala Lumpur, Malaysia.)

> "My hCG was measured from spinal fluid, which required a lumbar puncture. The lumbar puncture was absolutely the worst thing that I have ever had happen to me. I had to have two because they didn't draw off enough fluid in the first one. The doctor who tried to do the second had obviously not done many before (if any at all) and he stabbed around for ages not being able to get through before they had to sedate me, and get someone else to do it. I had terrible headaches for about two weeks afterwards." (Diagnosed at 30 in 1997; treated in Sheffield, UK.)

"Just a blood test...not a big deal" (Diagnosed at 32 in 2000; treated in Ontario, Canada.)

In very rare cases, some women may experience false positives when their hCG is tested by drawing blood. These women may have antibodies in their blood that interact with the hCG to produce a false positive, known as "phantom hCG." Women who have worked in a veterinary clinic, animal laboratory or zoo, and women who were raised on a farm are more likely to have the kinds of antibodies that may interfere with serum hCG tests. If there is any uncertainty, your healthcare provider should confirm that the hCG is a true value. The level of hCG found in your urine is unaffected by these antibodies, so if a blood test is positive for hCG but the urine test is negative, it is likely a false positive result.

Tests for Liver Enzymes and Kidney Function (Serum Chemistries)

Because chemotherapy drugs can affect the functioning of the liver and kidneys, blood chemistry is checked to make sure that these organs are functioning at an acceptable level. This blood test does not look for GTN or choriocarcinoma; rather, it looks at whether your liver and kidneys are healthy, because if they are then treatment can begin. If they're not healthy your doctor may decide to postpone treatment, or may choose a different course of therapy. Your doctor will continue to monitor your liver and kidney function throughout your treatment. If these organs aren't functioning properly your doctor will delay or stop chemotherapy for the time being.

Here is what one of the women we interviewed said about serum chemistries:

"Serum chemistries tons of times...I can't even remember how many 'cause they would give me this test every time I went to the emergency room, which was a lot before I was diagnosed." (Diagnosed at 24 in 2001; treated in New York City, NY.)

Complete Blood Count (CBC)

This test counts the number of blood cells of different types that are present in the bloodstream. A red blood cell count tells your doctor how much cell depletion has occurred because of uterine bleeding. The term "hematocrit" refers to the percentage of blood that is composed of red blood cells; for women this ranges from 35 to 45 percent. If your hematocrit is lower than this, you may be experiencing red blood cell depletion due to bleeding.

Your doctor will continue to measure your blood cell counts throughout your entire treatment. Chemotherapy can affect the white blood cells that are needed to fight infection. So, your doctor will want to monitor your level of white blood cells to be sure that you can still fight off any illness that might come your way. Chemotherapy can also affect the blood platelets that are needed for blood clotting. Blood clotting is essential for healing (this is what forms scabs), so these blood elements need to be carefully monitored.

Again, the CBC does not detect choriocarcinoma; rather, it detects the effect that chemotherapy is having on your blood. If your platelets or hematocrit (red blood cell percentage) are low, your doctor will schedule you for a blood transfusion. He or she may also recommend shots of a hormone called erythropoietin, which will help boost your bone marrow to make more red blood cells (this is described on pages 116–117). And if your white blood cells are low, you can either delay chemotherapy until your body produces more, or you can give yourself an injection of Neupogen® to produce more white blood cells, also described later on (see pages 112–115).

STAGING SYSTEMS FOR GTN

Once your doctor has received the results from all these tests, he or she will assess them, and then assign a stage to your GTN. Staging GTN measures the extent of the disease and the level of risk that is associated with the disease. The staging system combines information gained through diagnostic tests with our knowledge about risk factors for GTN (see page 33). Staging GTN helps the doctor to determine which treatment or chemotherapy protocol will be right for your particular disease given its unique features.

Until recently, doctors treating GTN utilized three different staging systems. The three systems used similar criteria to evaluate a patient's disease, but yielded very different stages and risk assessments. The World Health Organization (WHO) system evaluated several risk factors in order to assign cases of GTN to high- and low-risk categories. These risk categories helped physicians make treatment decisions. On the other hand, the International Federation of Gynecology and Obstetrics (FIGO) system staged the GTN according to whether it had spread (e.g., "Stage I" was used to describe localized disease and "Stage IV," widely metastatic disease).

Unfortunately, these numerous staging and risk factor systems were problematic. It was impossible, for example, to compare data on treatment efficacy from different centers. If a patient moved or chan{ often found that her staging score changed as well! The methods also made it difficult to compare clinical trials, which slowⅬⅬ the progress of finding new or improved treatments for GTN. In 2000, several GTN experts got together to discuss this problem. They consulted with numerous physicians involved in the management of GTN in order to develop a single, coherent staging system. All this hard work paid off and, in 2002, the International Federation of Gynecology and Obstetrics (FIGO) adopted a new classification system, which adapted all the best features of the three staging systems previously in use. However, since this system is relatively new, it isn't yet in use in all centers. You may want to ask your doctor about the staging system that he or she adheres to, and how it works.

We asked women with GTN if they knew what their score was. Surprisingly, most of the women we interviewed did not know their scores, or which staging system was used.

> "Was never informed of a particular stage. I had the full-blown disease. A tumor had ruptured on my kidney that lead to diagnosis." (Diagnosed at 41 in 2002; treated in Pensacola, Florida.)

> "In 1973, it was more or less [this] question: was the patient going to live or die? I don't think they even thought of it in stages." (Diagnosed at 27 in 1973; treated in Southampton, NY, and New York City, NY.)

> "I'm not sure what system was used, but I heard that I was stage 4 or 5...I can't remember." (Diagnosed at 32 in 2000; treated in Ontario, Canada.)

International Federation of Obstetrics and Gynecology (FIGO) 2000 Staging and Risk Factor Scoring System

The FIGO GTN classification system involves two measures. First, the doctor assigns a stage for the patient's GTN, and then the doctor calculates the patient's risk factors. This two-part system is represented by a Roman numeral (I, II, III, or IV) to indicate the stage of GTN; a colon, ":" to separate the two numbers; and an Arabic numeral (0–24) to represent the patient's risk factors. My classification number was III: 14; I will explain what these numbers mean once we take a closer look at the FIGO 2000 classification system.

First, let's look at the FIGO 2000 staging system. The doctor using this system orders several tests to determine the extent of your GTN. You may be asked to undergo a chest X-ray to see whether you GTN has spread to the lungs. You may have an ultrasound to determine whether you have metastases in your liver. You may receive a CT scan to find out whether there is GTN tissue in your lung, liver, brain or abdominal area. Finally you may receive an MRI to determine whether there are metasteses in your brain. These tests all provide slightly different information about the tumor, so your doctor may suggest that you have more than one of these tests. By looking at where (if anywhere) the GTN has spread, your doctor can then tell you the stage of your GTN.

Table 4.1: The FIGO 2000 Staging System

FIGO STAGING OF GTN	
Stage I	GTN is confined to the uterus
Stage II	GTN is found outside the uterus, but is limited to the genial structures (adnexa, vagina, broad ligament)
Stage III	GTN is found in the lungs (with or without genital tract involvement)
Stage IV	GTN is found in any other metastatic sites

Table reprinted with permission from: Dr. Ernest I. Kohorn (2003) "The FIGO 2000 Staging and Risk Factor Scoring System for Gestational Trophoblastic Neoplasia." Gestational Trophoblastic Disease 2nd Edition. B. W. Hancock, E. S. Newlands, R. S. Berkowitz and L. A. Cole (eds.) International Society for the Study of Trophoblastic Disease (ISSTD) www.isstd.org/gtd/index.html.

My GTN was stage III because I had GTN in my uterus and metastases in my lungs, but GTN tissue was not found anywhere else.

Next, we'll look at the FIGO 2000 risk factor scoring values. The number that your doctor calculates as your risk factor will put you in either the high-risk or the low-risk category. Once your doctor knows your risk-value he or she will be able to better prepare a plan for treating your GTN. To determine your risk-value your doctor will ask you a series of questions about things such as your age, whether you've had chemotherapy before, your experience with the pregnancy that lead to GTN, and how long it's been since you were pregnant (unless, of course you are still pregnant). The last question about the time interval since pregnancy allows the doctor to estimate how long the GTN tissue has been present in your body. The doctor will order blood tests to measure the level of hCG in your bloodstream. The amount of hCG present in the bloodstream estimates the overall extent of the GTN tissue present in your body. Your doctor will also examine the imaging tests (CT, MRI, X-ray or ultrasound) to estimate the size of the largest tumor. Once this is done, your doctor will compare your information to the table below and calculate a risk factor.

Table 4.2: The FIGO 2000 Risk Factor Scoring Values

RISK FACTORS	SCORE ASSIGNED TO THE RISK FACTORS			
	0	1	2	4
Woman's Age	< 40	>40		
Preceding Pregnancy	Hydatidi-form Mole	Abortion	Term	
Months Since Preceding Pregnancy	<4	4 – <7	7 – <13	≥13
Pre-treatmen hCG (IU/liter)	<1,000 ($< 10^3$)	1,000- 10,000 (10^3-10^4)	10,000- 100,000 (10^4-10^5)	> 100,000 (>10^5)
Largest Tumor (including original Uterine Tumor)	< 3 cm	3 – < 5 cm	≥ 5 cm	
Site of Metastases	Lung	Spleen Kidney	GI Tract Liver	Brain
Number of Metastases Identified		1 – 4	5 – 8	> 8
Prior Chemotherapy			Single Drug	2 or more Drugs
The total score for a patient is obtained by adding the individual scores for each prognostic factor. Then, the risk category can be determined. Scoring: ≤ 6 = low risk; ≥ 7 = high risk.				

73

Table on previous page reprinted with permission from: Dr. Ernest I. Kohorn (2003) "The FIGO 2000 Staging and Risk Factor Scoring System for Gestational Trophoblastic Neoplasia." Gestational Trophoblastic Disease 2nd Edition. B. W. Hancock, E. S. Newlands, R. S. Berkowitz and L. A. Cole (eds.) International Society for the Study of Trophoblastic Disease (ISSTD) www.isstd.org/gtd/index.html.

My Risk factor value was 14. Here is how it was calculated:

MY RISK FACTOR	SCORE
My Age at diagnosis: **< 40**	0
My pregnancy preceding the GTN: **term**	2
Time between my pregnancy and diagnosis with GTN: **9 months**	2
My hCG level at diagnosis: **556,000 IU/liter**	4
My largest tumor: **8 cm**	2
Site of my metastases: **lungs only**	0
Total number of metstases they counted for me: **12**	4
I had never had chemotherapy before	0
MY TOTAL SCORE	14

The new FIGO 2000 staging and risk factor scoring system gives standardized and accurate classification for patients with GTN. The risk assessment allows your doctor to properly plan your treatment (see chapter 5). However, the system is not perfect and has a few drawbacks. The two main drawbacks are that two forms of GTN remain outside this classification system. First, there is no means for assessing molar pregnancies that do not progress to GTN. Second, placental site trophoblastic tumors (PSTT) cannot be classified on the FIGO 2000 system. Some physicians have considered adding a stage "0" to the classification system to deal with molar pregnancies, but it remains unclear what to do about PSTT.

HOW TO DEAL WITH DOCTORS AND YOUR HEALTHCARE TEAM

Before you were diagnosed with GTN or choriocarcinoma, chances are you probably didn't have too much contact with doctors. After your diagnosis, your relationship with the medical profession changes dramatically. Suddenly, doctors are a part of your daily life. It stands to reason that the care you receive from these doctors will make a huge difference in terms of your chances of survival, so it pays to develop a good relationship with them. I was seriously overlooked and put on the back burner by my OBGYN before being diagnosed with choriocarcinoma. Then, once I was already receiving care for choriocarcinoma, I decided to switch gynecological oncologists. I did this because Dr. A resisted answering even the most basic questions. I asked him what was being put in my IV, for example, and his reply was "one of the chemo drugs." I then rephrased the question, and asked what the drug was called. He just repeated his answer. I asked if I would feel any immediate side effects from the chemo and his answer was that everyone reacts differently to chemo. Clearly, his answers weren't helpful at all.

Furthermore, he treated me like a child. He answered many of my questions by being short and evasive—as if he were talking to a two year-old child. For example, I'd been having very sharp back pain and throbbing in my lower back (almost like a migraine, but in the lower back area instead). So I mentioned this to him and he told me that it was just from "every day wear and tear." I'd actually researched this type of pain and discovered it was one of the side effects of an injection I had to get to bring my white blood cell (WBC) count up. I'd also asked him, when I got my blood checked, what certain things mean (hemoglobin, WBC, CBC, creatinine, platelets, etc.). His reply, in a patronizing tone of voice, was: "why do you need to know that?"

I told Dr. A that I didn't want the resident looking after me anymore. The doctor didn't listen, and the next day the resident came in to see me again. I was so mad! TJ later stopped the doctor in the hall and told him that I didn't want the resident treating me. Dr. A said, "Oh, she's just being a woman." Which meant that not only was my doctor ignoring my requests, he had a sexist attitude to boot! I didn't think his way of handling things (or me) was the right way, but it wasn't until later that I found out I could refuse treatment from him. I didn't know I had a choice.

As the patient it's your right to decide who should treat you (where there *is* a choice) and how much involvement you want to have in your care. You have the right to ask questions and have them answered honestly. You also have the right to change your mind about your level of involvement *at any time* during the course of your treatment. If you feel tired and you don't want to think about the complex issues involved in cancer treatment, you can tell your doctor that you want him or her to decide on these issues for you. You can also elect to have a loved one or a friend decide. Forcing information on patients is as detrimental as keeping patients in the dark. For more information on this and issues like this, please see the American Hospital Association's "Patient's Bill of Rights" located on this webpage: *www.patienttalk.info/AHA-Patient_Bill_of_Rights.htm.*

How to Choose Your Doctor

In many cases, there's little "choice" involved in your choice of doctor. GTN and choriocarcinoma are very rare, so in smaller cities especially there are often few doctors with experience in treating it. During the course of my chorio treatment I moved from Toronto, Ontario (a city of 4 million) to Saskatoon, Saskatchewan (a city of 200,000). I decided to move because I felt the need to be around all my family and friends back home. When I discussed this with my second gynecological oncologist—let's call him Dr. "B"; he was much kinder than the Dr. A I describe above—he was concerned I wouldn't get the best care here in Saskatoon. In Saskatoon a regular oncologist (as opposed to one who specializes in gynecological cancers) treated me—let's call her Dr. "C." She frequently conversed with the gynecological oncologist from Toronto (Dr. B), which made me feel better.

You should look for a gynecological oncologist who has experience in treating choriocarcinoma. If there isn't anyone with experience in your area be sure that your doctor has a specialist with whom he or she can consult on your treatment. It's also important to find a doctor with whom you feel comfortable. You'll have to share some pretty sensitive information with this person, so you should feel comfortable discussing everything about your treatment (as well as aspects of your sexual well-being and lifestyle, such as smoking and drug use). You should also be able to discuss complementary medicines, such as herbal supplements, if you feel inclined to take these. If possible, try to sit down and have a conversation with a few prospective doctors to see how you feel about each one of them.

Some Tips for Choosing Your Doctor

1. You don't have to go to the first doctor who was recommended. Find out about the doctors and clinics in your area that offer care for patients with GTN and choriocarcinoma.

2. Take a look at the questions at the end of this chapter (especially those regarding credentials and experience, as well as a few others of interest to you) and then sit down with prospective doctors and ask them to answer these questions. Pay attention to the way the doctor answers each one. Does the doctor seem to have enough time for you? Can you trust this doctor? Do you like the way he or she talks to you and pays attention to you? Do you feel that you're getting the very best answer this doctor is capable of giving? Are you confident that if this doctor didn't know the answer to one of your questions, he or she would do everything possible to get it?

3. Because of confidentiality issues it is not always possible to speak with other patients, but you may want to ask your doctor whether any patients have volunteered to be resources for new patients. If so, consider talking to other patients receiving care from this doctor. Also talk to patients who switched out of this doctor's care, if possible. Ask about their reasons for switching. You might want to find out if the patient you're talking to wanted to know a lot or a little about her treatment. Think about whether this patient's desired level of involvement matches yours, and whether this has affected the perspective she brings to the quality of her care.

4. If possible, try to choose a doctor or treatment center that's in your neighborhood. The treatment for GTN can be quite lengthy. You may need to make multiple visits and so you may want to choose a doctor near your home. This isn't always possible, but it should be a consideration.

Warning Signs and Red Flags

Even if you thought that a particular doctor was a good match at the outset, you may find that your feelings change during the course of treatment. If this happens, don't hesitate to speak up and try to resolve the situation. The first approach may be to discuss the matter with your doctor. Let him or her know that you have concerns about your ability to communicate openly. Even if you feel very frustrated or angry, it's better to avoid being hostile or accusatory toward your doctor. People will often become defensive and withdraw if they feel attacked. The American Cancer Society has a good webpage entitled "Talking with Your Doctor" can be searched for here: *www.cancer.org/.*

But if talking to your doctor doesn't work, if you're too frustrated to remain calm or talking seems too intimidating, you can try talking to another member of the hospital staff. There are nurses, social workers, bioethicists and patient representatives whose job it is to help mediate communications and complaints between patients and their physicians. Sometimes this is less stressful than confronting your doctor directly.

If these approaches don't work, it may be time to find a new doctor. Never stay with a doctor just to protect his or her feelings. *You have the right to request a transfer to another doctor if there is one available.* The "last straw" that signaled to me it was time to switch doctors was when my first gynecologic oncologist, Dr A, asked me if I was taking birth control, and what kind. Since he'd performed my hysterectomy, I thought he should know that I wasn't using birth control. I felt that he really didn't care about me as a person or as a patient.

When to Switch Doctors

- You bring up a problem, a question or a concern and nothing changes.
- The doctor or clinic makes the same mistake more than once.
- Your doctor makes you feel stupid or inadequate.
- Your doctor makes you feel judged.
- Your doctor is condescending or patronizing.
- The doctor leaves your questions unanswered. (Your doctor has a duty to fully answer all of your questions in a language you understand.)
- Your doctor does not inform you of all your options for treatment and expected side effects.
- You feel that the lack of trust between you and your doctor is interfering with your care.

- You can't open up to your doctor.
- You find another doctor who has experience in choriocarcinoma and appears to offer more of what you need in terms of convenience, sensitivity and/or better care.

Adapted from Sandra Trisdale "Working with your Doctor" WORLD: 3, April 2002 and the Canadian Cancer Society booklet "Taking Time."

Patient Responsibilities

Doctors have certain responsibilities regarding their patients, but it's important to remember that patients have responsibilities regarding their treatment as well. You have the responsibility to make all of your appointments—unless you have a really good reason for missing one. If you do have to miss an appointment, call your doctor to cancel. This allows other patients to use your appointment time. If there are any barriers to your healthcare (you can't find a ride to and from your chemotherapy appointments, or you can't find childcare, or your medications are too expensive, or you've lost your job and can't pay your rent) let your doctor know. He or she may know of an assistance program, or may be able to refer you to a social worker or case manager who can help.

Before you go to your doctor's, make a list of the symptoms you're experiencing. Try to state as clearly as possible any changes in your body functions, including sleep, bowel habits and headaches. No complaint is too small, as it might signal a further problem. And if side effects are making your life miserable, let your doctor know. There may be other treatment options.

Treat yourself with respect. Don't neglect your health to take care of others. This may be easier said than done if you have a new baby to care for, but please do try to get some help and some rest. Your loved ones need you yet the best you can do for them is to concentrate on healing. For more information, please see the American Hospital Association's "Patient's Bill of Responsibilities" webpage: *www.patienttalk.info/AHA-Patient_Bill_of_Rights.htm.*

QUESTIONS TO ASK YOUR DOCTOR

Different questions are important at different stages in your treatment. Some questions will come up repeatedly, as your situation changes. Don't be afraid to ask your doctor the same question on more than one occasion.

Many patients find it difficult to absorb all the information that their doctor is telling them. For this reason, it's a good idea to bring along a tape recorder, if you have one, to record the doctor's answers. Alternatively, you can bring a family member or friend along to jot down the answers or make notes on your behalf. That way it will be easy to remember what the doctor advised. If something seemed clear when the doctor first explained it, but now seems confusing, don't be afraid to ask about it again. The information concerning a diagnosis as complex as GTN often needs to be repeated several times.

Here is a list of questions we compiled from various sources. You may not feel like asking all of these questions on the first visit. However, you can refer back to this list on subsequent visits to see if any of the questions now seem more relevant.

Questions About Your Doctor's Credentials and Experience
- Where did you earn your MD?
- Have you had fellowship training in oncology (specifically, gynecologic oncology) and if so where?
- How long have you been practicing?
- How many cases of GTN have you treated in the past? How many cases are you currently treating?
- What have been the outcomes for the patients with GTN who you have treated in the past?

General Questions
- What kind of gestational trophoblastic neoplasia do I have?
- Based on what you've learned about my disease, do you think it can be cured?
- Has my disease spread beyond my uterus? If so, where has it spread?
- What is the stage and prognostic classification of my disease? What staging system are you using (see pages 70–74 for more details)?

Questions About Treatment

- Are there other treatment options?
- How long will it take me to recover from treatment?
- How should I expect to feel during treatment?
- Should I get a second opinion?
- What are the risks and benefits of these treatments?
- What is all the bloodwork for? What is measured?
- What should I do to be ready for treatment?
- What side effects, if any, can I expect to have?
- What tests are involved in all of this?
- What treatment choices do I have?
- What treatments do you recommend?
- When can I go back to work after treatment?
- What medicines are you giving me? What are they for?

Questions About Recurrence

- Does one type of treatment reduce the risk of recurrence more than another?
- What are the chances that my cancer will recur?

Questions About Your Healthcare Team

- Can my family members talk to you or another member of my healthcare team if they have any questions? (You will also have to let your doctor know which family members are allowed information on your health status, since health confidentiality is protected by law.)
- When can I call you if I have a question?
- What situations warrant a call to my doctor? Which signs should I look out for and which need to be reported right away?
- Who can I call if I have a concern after hours?
- Who else gets information about me? Who has access to my medical records?
- Will a specialist in gynecologic oncology (a specialist in cancers of the female reproductive organs) be involved in my care?
- Will my case be used to educate medical students and/or residents at this facility? Do I have the right to refuse to participate in this education?

Questions About Lifestyle and Treatment

- Can I have a glass of wine or a drink while I am receiving treatments?
- How soon after treatment can I have sex?
- How soon after treatment can I get pregnant?
- What are my prospects of having a normal pregnancy later on?

CHAPTER 5

TREATING GTN AND CHORIOCARCINOMA

There are three basic ways to fight GTN: surgery, chemotherapy and radiation therapy. Surgery and chemotherapy are the most common treatments used in fighting GTN. Radiation therapy is rarely used to treat GTN, so we will not deal with it in this book. If your doctor suggests radiation therapy you can contact your local cancer society to ask them for information. Exactly which treatments are chosen depends on many things, including the center where your GTN is being treated, the type of GTN that you have, and where (if anywhere) the GTN has spread. If cells from the placenta have traveled to other organs, then treatment may be more complicated (and it may be necessary to use more than one type of treatment).

In my case, I had a D&C, three different regimens of the combination chemotherapy as well as a hysterectomy. All of them had different physical and emotional side effects. But people have different experiences and are affected by the same things in different ways. For me, it was quite tough. I found that after a few months the chemo affected me more and more. After a while it got to the point where I didn't feel like myself. I wasn't able to do many of the things I enjoyed doing because I was so weak, and because I felt sick all the time.

I can remember one day when I had enough energy to get out of bed and was able to stay on the couch, but wasn't able to do much else. My daughter Tatum was doing something really cute and funny. All I could do was lie there. At the time, I thought: I should be laughing at this, but I don't have the energy or the willpower to do it. That absolutely killed me inside. I know she was too young at the time to remember, but it still hurts to think that this was how I had to live my life. It got a lot better after that. My chemotherapy protocol eventually changed, and I found this last one (taxol, cisplatin and etopiside) to be less harsh for side effects, which allowed me to get my energy back up again. I wasn't so sick all the time, and I quickly gained back the weight I had lost.

TREATMENTS BY TYPE AND STAGE OF GTN

This section discusses the standard treatments that are used in cases of GTN. They'll likely be similar to the treatments that you receive, but they may not be exactly the same, since your doctor may decide to treat your unique disease in a unique way, a way that's designed just for you. Furthermore, treatment varies from one region to the next, so if you hear something from a friend or family member that's different than what's happening to you, you don't need to be alarmed. (Although you may want to ask your doctor to explain why he or she is doing things differently.)

The type of treatment used will depend on the form and stage of your gestational trophoblastic neoplasia. The treatment for moles often involves surgery alone. Sometimes chemotherapy will be used to treat moles, especially if the mole is persistent. Low-risk choriocarcinoma is usually treated using only one chemotherapy drug, perhaps combined with surgery. High-risk choriocarcinoma is treated using a combination of chemotherapy drugs, and sometimes requires surgery. Recurrent GTN is automatically placed in a high-risk category, simply because it has recurred. Recurrent GTN is therefore treated with a combination of chemotherapy drugs, sometimes along with surgery and radiation therapy as well. And if the disease has spread to other areas in the body, these areas may also be treated with surgery or radiation therapy.

The women we interviewed told us how long it took from the time of diagnosis to the time they went into remission:

> "I was diagnosed July 19, 2001, was cancer free by November 20, 2001, and had chemo to February 20, 2002. Which is pretty good considering my hCG was 9.5 million when diagnosed." (Diagnosed at 24 in 2001; treated in New York City, NY.)

> "Diagnosis: August 1993. Remission: June 1999." (Diagnosed at 36 in 1993; treated in Manila, Philippines and Kuala Lumpur, Malaysia.)

> "It was 18 months from diagnosis to hysterectomy (which my doctor now considers my cure point) but [I had] another 2 months of EMACO, so you could say 20 months." (Diagnosed at 41 in 1999; Treated in Memphis, TN, then Fort Lauderdale, FL.)

"I would say that my treatment lasted a total of four months from D&C to release from Sloan Kettering. However, my tests lasted a couple of years longer." (Diagnosed at 27 in 1973; treated in Southampton, NY and New York City, NY.)

Hydatidiform Mole

Once the diagnosis is made, the hydatidiform mole is removed by suction curettage or by dilation and curettage (D&C) in the operating room under anesthesia (see pages 90–92 for more on D&Cs). If you've finished with childbearing, your doctor may recommend a hysterectomy rather than a D&C (see pages 95–100 for the advantages and disadvantages of hysterectomy).

Once the mole has been removed by D&C, the amount of hCG in your blood may lower to normal levels (0–5). If this happens, no further treatment will be required, and your doctor will simply monitor your blood samples for any reoccurrence. However, if the amount of hCG in your blood samples does not lower, rises for two weeks, or plateaus for more than three weeks, then chemotherapy may be administered.

In approximately one third of women with a molar pregnancy, there may be one or more cysts on one or both ovaries. The cysts are caused by high levels of hCG. In the majority of cases, these cysts don't need to be removed, as they disappear on their own. Sometimes the cysts can rupture, bleed or become infected, in which case they may need to be removed (an ovarian cystectomy is removal of the ovarian cyst, whereas an oophorectomy is removal of the ovary). You should discuss these possibilities with your doctor before you head into the operating room, especially if the recommended operation is a hysterectomy (removal of the uterus).

Complications associated with the treatment of hydatidiform mole include: anemia due to blood loss, severe high blood pressure, an overactive thyroid gland, heart failure, hemorrhage, infection and acute pulmonary failure.

The survival rate for women with a hydatidiform mole, whether treated with surgery alone, or with surgery and chemotherapy, is nearly 100 percent.

Non-Metastatic GTN (Invasive Mole, Persistent Mole and Non-Metastatic Choriocarcinoma)

Non-metastatic GTN is either an invasive mole or choriocarcinoma. Non-metastatic GTN simply means that the placental cells haven't spread to other organs of the body and that there is no disease outside of the uterus. All cases of non-metastatic GTN are considered curable, even if there is extensive disease in the uterus. Treatment usually begins with chemotherapy and, if this fails, a hysterectomy is performed.

The standard chemotherapy for non-metastatic disease is usually a single chemotherapy drug, often methotrexate if your liver is healthy and in good shape (for more details on methotrexate see the B.C. Cancer Agency Drug Manual or CancerBACUP Chemotherapy Drug Manual, listed in the resources at the back of this book). If your liver function is poor then actinomycin-D is used (for more information on actinomycin-D see the B.C. Cancer Agency Drug Manual or CancerBACUP Chemotherapy Drug Manual, listed in the resources at the back of this book).

There are several ways that methotrexate can be administered. Often it is taken daily (by injection or IV) for 5 days. Then you're given a 14-day rest and recovery period. The 5 days of injection plus the recovery period are known as a "cycle." Your blood is monitored and this cycle is repeated until you hCG returns to normal. It usually takes 3 to 4 cycles to achieve remission.

Alternatively, methotrexate may be administered with leucovorin rescue. In this case the cycle is 8 days long. Methotrexate is administered on days 1, 3, 5 and 7; and leucovorin is given on days 2, 4, 6 and 8. When given in this way, usually only one course of treatment is required (with a remission rate of about 80 percent). A third way to give the methotrexate is weekly. If the hCG levels in your blood do not return to normal, then a second or even third course may be given.

Actinomycin-D is usually given intravenously for five consecutive days. This cycle is repeated every two weeks. Actinomycin-D may also be given in a larger dose on a single day, and this cycle will be repeated every two weeks until the level of hCG in your blood returns to normal. If actinomycin-D does not produce a remission, then your doctor will probably decide to change to methotrexate.

The survival rate for non-metastatic GTN (both invasive moles and non-metastatic choriocarcinoma) is nearly 100 percent.

Low-Risk Metastatic GTN (Metastatic Mole and Metastatic Choriocarcinoma)

Metastatic choriocarcinoma is considered low risk when:

- it's diagnosed less than four months after the onset of the pregnancy;
- the hCG count is low;
- there are no tumors in the liver or brain; and
- the patient has had no previous chemotherapy.

Please see pages 70–74 for more information on risk categories.

The standard treatment for low-risk metastatic GTN is usually a single chemotherapy drug (see non-metastatic GTN, previous). If single agent treatment fails, which happens about 20 percent of the time, the doctor will enlist a combination of chemotherapy drugs. However, some physicians prefer to *begin* with a combination of chemotherapy drugs. In this case a doctor administers both methotrexate and actinomycin-D, sometimes in conjunction with cyclophosphamide as well (called MA or MAC for short). The drug combination is given for five consecutive days every two to three weeks until the patient's hCG returns to normal.

The survival rate for low-risk metastatic GTN is 97 to 100 percent.

High-Risk Metastatic GTN (Metastatic Mole and Metastatic Choriocarcinoma)

Metastatic GTN is considered high risk when:

- it's diagnosed more than four months after the onset of the pregnancy;
- the hCG count is high;
- there are tumors in the liver or brain;
- the patient has had prior chemotherapy; or
- the GTN occurred after a full-term pregnancy

Please see pages 70–74 for more information on risk categories.

High-risk GTN must be treated as soon as possible after diagnosis with an aggressive, multiple-agent chemotherapy course. If there are tumors in the brain or liver, treatment will often involve radiation therapy to those areas.

In the past, treatment used for high-risk metastatic GTN was called CHAMOCA. This regimen used hydroxyurea, actinomycin-D, methotrexate, folinic acid, cyclophosphamide, vincristin and doxorubicin. This form of treatment had a success rate of about 76 percent. Another old form of treatment was called CHAMOMA, which added melphan to the drugs listed above. This treatment produced remission 82 percent of the time. These therapies were harsh on the body. The side effects were so intense that the patient often needed long breaks between treatments in order to recover enough to receive the next dose. Unfortunately, the cancer cells were able to recover in that time as well. This meant that treatments lasted a long time. The Charing Cross Hospital in London, England recognized that a new course of therapy was required for these patients. Doctors there developed a new therapy, which has now become the standard for treating high-risk metastatic GTN.

Standard treatment now involves a mixture of chemotherapeutic agents that include etoposide, methotrexate, actinomycin-D, vincristine and cyclophosphamide (EMA-CO for short). Sometimes cisplatin and etoposide are used instead of vincristine and cyclophosphamide (and in this case the treatment is referred to as EMA-CE or EP-EMA). Your doctor will work out the exact details of your treatment, according to your overall health. Fortunately, this new course of treatment doesn't usually require long breaks for recovery time, unless your white blood cell (WBC) count has fallen too low. The invention of drugs called granulocyte colony stimulating factor (G-CSF, such as Neupogen®) that act to raise WBC counts, has further decreased the need for breaks.

The survival rate for high-risk metastatic GTN is between 75 and 86 percent. A study conducted at the Charing Cross hospital in England reported that among patients, no deaths occurred later than two years after starting the EMA-CO regimen. So if you've made it two years, you're probably in the clear!

I was categorized as high risk. When I learned of the survival rate my heart started jumping and my breath basically stopped. I was terrified, and to this day even thinking about it still affects me in this way. But, all I could do was hope for the best and make myself one of that 75 percent. I thought, "I won't let this cancer beat me. I have too much living to do to die now."

New studies conducted at the GTN center in Sheffield recently reported a success rate of 85 percent using a chemotherapy regimen that combines methotrexate, etoposide and actinomycin-D alone (called MEA for short). This treatment is easier on the patient and may soon become the standard therapy for high-risk metastatic GTN patients. (It's currently being adopted as the standard in Japan.)

Metastatic GTN that Includes Metastases in the Central Nervous System

Patients who have metastases in the brain are usually treated with one of the high-risk protocols mentioned above. They're also often treated with radiation therapy to reduce the risk of brain hemorrhage. Radiation therapy is sometimes accompanied by brain surgery in selected cases. The cure rate for this form of treatment is still quite high, around 86 percent.

Placental Site Trophoblastic Tumors (PSTT)

Placental site trophoblastic tumors don't usually metastasize. Non-metastatic PSTT is treated with surgery, either D&C or hysterectomy. Metastatic PSTT is treated using etoposide and cisplatin one week; and etoposide, methotrexate and actinomycin-D the following week (called EP-EMA for short). However, since metastasis with PSTT is so rare, the optimum therapy is not well studied.

The survival rate for patients with PSTT is about 15 to 20 percent in those with metastatic disease. However, the survival rate may be improved by including cisplatin in the initial treatment.

CHEMOTHERAPY RESISTANCE

Sometimes the cancer cells become resistant to treatment with the first-line chemotherapy regimen that a patient is prescribed. It's as though the cancer cells have become "used to" the chemotherapy. If this happens then a new treatment protocol is developed using different chemotherapeutic drugs. The second line of treatment chosen depends upon the level of hCG (when resistance developed) and the initial stage of gestational trophoblastic neoplasia. Even when chemotherapy resistance occurs, most patients respond to a change in the chemotherapy regimen (for more on chemotherapy resistance please see chapter 8).

Low-Risk Patients with Chemotherapy Resistance

Low-risk patients who develop chemotherapy resistance when their hCG is at or below 100 iu/L receive single-agent chemotherapy using actinomycin-D. This is administered every day for five days, followed by two days rest, and the course of treatment is repeated for two weeks. This treatment achieves remission in 86.6 percent of low-risk patients with chemotherapy resistance. If that fails (which can occur in 13.4 percent of patients with chemotherapy resistance), the physician may decide to switch the patient to a combination of chemotherapy drugs. Usually the physician will decide to use either the EMA-CO or the EMA-EP regimen.

Low-risk patients who develop resistance to their treatment when their hCG is more than 100 iu/L are given a combination of chemotherapy agents. Often it's the EMA-CO regime, which consists of etopiside, methotrexate and actinomycin-D one week, and cyclophosphamide and vincristine the second week. This regime has resulted in a 98.9 percent success rate in resistant patients.

High-Risk Patients with Chemotherapy Resistance

High-risk patients who develop a resistance to the first-line EMA-CO regimen are switched to a combination of chemotherapy drugs that includes etopiside and cisplatin one week, and etopiside, methotrexate and actinomycin-D the second week (called EP-EMA). Seventy percent of patients who received this form of treatment after developing a resistance to EMA-CO experienced a complete remission. Some scientists feel that this treatment should be the first used for patients with ultra-high-risk GTN. It hasn't yet become standard therapy, however, since the ultra-high-risk category has only recently been added to the WHO staging system. Ultra-high-risk patients are those who have multiple high-risk factors, such as a term pregnancy or metastases in the brain or liver.

TREATMENT FOLLOW-UP

Once your hCG counts have returned to normal (which can be anywhere from 0 to 5 mIU/mL) then your treatment will be considered successful. Your doctor will still want to continue to monitor the amount of hCG in your blood. He or she will ask you to make a bloodwork appointment once a week for the first 4 to 14 weeks after your counts reach normal. Then you'll have monthly appointments for six months to a year. After this first year your doctor will monitor your blood once every six months for the following three years (for molar pregnancies or low-risk GTN the monitoring period may be considerably shorter).

You'll be advised to use a reliable method of birth control for a year after your treatment is finished. This is because a normal, healthy pregnancy will raise your levels of hCG, and will make it difficult for your doctor to tell if the increase is due to pregnancy, or to the return of GTN. However, after this initial period, you should be able to get pregnant again (see chapter 9 for more on pregnancy after GTN).

Some of the women we spoke to told us about their treatment follow-up:

> "I used to get really nervous when I went for a follow-up, hoping that everything would be alright. But now I'm getting used to it and I'm glad that my follow-ups are the way they are. I'm very comfortable with them." (Diagnosed at 24 in 2001; Treated in New York City, NY.)

> "Immediately after stopping treatment I was very apprehensive about not having chemo anymore and couldn't quite believe that it was going to work and I wouldn't be going back [to the hospital] again." (Diagnosed at 30 in 1997; treated in Sheffield, UK.)

> "I was monitored very closely due to my recurrences. I had weekly bloodwork, hCG and CBC (since my white cell counts were shot) for 13 weeks, then every 2 weeks until the 9-month mark or so, then every 3 weeks until a year post-chemo, then every month. I still get labs every 6 weeks, just for my own peace of mind. I see my doctor every 3 months, but at my 2-year mark (which will be August) I'l stop going!" (Diagnosed at 41 in 1999; treated in Memphis, TN then Fort Lauderdale, FL.)

Some Questions You May Want to Ask Your Doctor about Your Follow-Up Care

- How often do I need to return for checkups?
- Do I need more X-rays, scans or blood tests? Why do I need these? What will they tell me?
- Will I need more chemotherapy, surgery, radiation therapy or another type of treatment?
- How will I know when I'm cured? What are the chances that the cancer will come back?
- How soon can I go back to my regular activities (work, sex, sports)?

- Do I need to take any special precautions?
- Do I need to follow a special diet?

Recurrent GTN

In rare instances GTN will recur. This happens in about 2.5 percent of women with non-metastatic disease, 3.7 percent of women with low-risk metastatic disease and 13 percent of women with high-risk metastatic disease. Almost all recurrences take place within three years of remission (85 percent recur in the first 18 months). However, sometimes GTN may reoccur a long time after that, even after a normal, full-term pregnancy.

Recurrent disease is usually treated with chemotherapy (the same course as in high-risk GTN, described above). See chapter 8 for more on recurrent GTN.

GTN TREATMENT PARTICULARS: SURGERY

Surgery is an important tool in treating GTN. The goal of surgery is to physically remove as much of the placental tissue as possible. Sometimes it's necessary to use chemotherapy or radiation therapy to shrink the overgrown placenta to a more manageable size before surgery is performed. Other times it's necessary to undergo chemotherapy after surgery to ensure that even placental cells that may have been missed by surgery are treated.

Surgery is the most common form of treatment for GTN and choriocarcinoma. Nearly all GTN treatment begins with a D&C or suction curettage to remove any abnormal tissues.

Dilation & Curettage (D&C) and Suction Curettage

Dilation and curettage and suction curettage both refer to the surgical removal of the tissues that line the uterine wall. These are very common and low-risk types of surgery. In D&C the cervix is dilated sufficiently for the introduction of a sharp instrument, called a "curette," which scrapes away the contents of the uterus. In suction curettage, the same end is achieved by inserting a cannula (or small tube) into the cervix and applying suction to the cannula. Recent studies suggest that suction curettage is preferable to dilation and curettage. This is because the mole or tumor may have invaded deeply into the uterus, and it's easier to puncture the uterus with the metal curette. Both these operations can be performed under general or local anesthesia. Local anesthesia is more common however, and can be combined with pre-operative sedation.

As you now know, these surgeries remove the abnormal or cancerous placental cells from the uterus of patients with GTN. If the GTN is caught early, surgery may be enough to cure the GTN, or prevent the spread of placental cells to other organs. D&C has a very low complication rate: approximately one to four percent. The psychological effects of these operations are often the most difficult part.

Many of the women we interviewed had D&Cs as a part of their treatment for chorio:

> "I had two [D&Cs]. One when I was first diagnosed and one later when they thought the tumor was confined to inside the uterus. I had a general anesthetic. [I felt] upset at losing what I thought was a baby, and thinking: I hope this works and I don't die." (Diagnosed at 30 in 1997; treated in Sheffield, UK.)

> "I was nervous, as I'd never had surgery before, but figured many women had this, [and] they got through it OK. I was anxious to get rid of the foreign thing inside me. That night I was really tired and nauseous and had a lot of pills to take. I remember I couldn't wait to take my next pain pill (which is unusual since I pride myself on going "natural"). Two days later my husband took me for a drive just to get out of the townhouse, but after 15 minutes, all I wanted to do was sleep! I thought this [procedure] would get at the molar tissue, and I wasn't worried since my original OBGYN told me it would probably take care of things." (Diagnosed at 41 in 1999; treated in Memphis, TN, then Fort Lauderdale, FL.)

> "It was easy, with no post-operative pain whatsoever. I was under general anesthesia." (Diagnosed at 36 in 1993; treated in Manila, Philippines, and Kuala Lumpur, Malaysia.)

Emotions and the Loss of a Pregnancy

Having a D&C because your GTN indicates that there is a serious defect with your fetus increases your risk of experiencing a negative emotional and/or psychological response to the surgery. In many cases, the pregnancy was wanted. Some women feel that they're responsible for the fetus's defects. It's important to remember that GTN occurs because of random genetic mistakes (see chapter 2). Nothing that you ate, smoked, played or did during your pregnancy caused the GTN. There is *no way* to prevent GTN from occurring.

Women who lost babies they wanted report that they found little support for their emotions. Our culture often doesn't respond to or adequately support the various feelings of loss we experience. A woman may feel that she and her husband are the only two people who care about the loss at all. Sometimes husbands, who are trying to be supportive, are too strong. A woman may think her husband isn't feeling anything, because he's trying to ignore his own feelings in order to be supportive of her feelings. Women sometimes wish that their husbands would show emotion so they wouldn't feel like they're alone, or like they're overreacting to the situation.

I had a very emotional reaction to the D&C. And in my case, I didn't have the added stress of dealing with the loss of a wanted pregnancy. After the surgery, I woke up really drowsy, and had to sleep in the recovery room until the anesthesia wore off. When I was released I felt somewhat lost, cranky, tired, and very emotional. My body had gone through a lot, and most people didn't realize that. They thought that because I wasn't kept overnight in the hospital that it was an easy procedure, one that should've been a piece of cake. But it really took a lot out of me. I was tired to begin with, so I think that just added to it. I mostly slept and whined about things for the rest of the day!

Prospective fathers also experience a variety of emotional reactions to the loss of a pregnancy; however, prospective fathers tend to express these emotions differently. Prospective fathers have reported feeling like they've failed their wives and their lost child. They may feel they were inadequate in the role of provider and protector. A prospective father's attachment to the developing baby is often more abstract because he lacks the intense physical relationship experienced by the pregnant woman. One study reported that the intensity of the prospective father's grief was consistently less than that of the prospective mother. This may be because the baby is often more "real" to the pregnant woman than to the prospective father. Most prospective fathers who lost a child reported that the intensity of their feelings of loss was greater than they anticipated.

This sense of loss was especially acute for families who had already begun to prepare for the arrival of the new child. The more the baby had become a presence in the family's life, the more difficult it was to deal with the loss.

Fathers for whom the baby was real, those who had seen the ultrasound or heard the heartbeat, had a harder time dealing with the loss of the pregnancy.

One study of prospective fathers who had experienced a miscarriage found that many men expressed their grief by keeping busy and trying to "handle things" at the time of the loss. They busied themselves with caring for their other children, removing the baby furniture from the home, and dealing with telling their friends and family about the loss, so that their wife wouldn't have to. Prospective fathers also tried to make sure that their wives were feeling alright. This is often appreciated, but can sometimes make the wife feel that she is the only one who cared about the child. None of the fathers in the study complained about the amount of support that *they* received after the loss. They felt no need to discuss their feelings of loss with anyone other than their wives.

Hysterectomy

Hysterectomy refers to the surgical removal of the entire uterus (womb). There are many different types of hysterectomy procedures and you should ask your doctor which one you'll be receiving. A hysterectomy is usually a successful operation, but when you have GTN a hysterectomy can be a life-saving operation, too. About 15 percent of hysterectomies are performed to treat cancer of the uterus, ovaries or cervix. If you've completed your child-bearing then a hysterectomy might be recommended straightaway. The advantage of a hysterectomy in this case is that most of the placental cells will be located in the uterus, since this is where the GTN or choriocarcinoma began. The disadvantage is that, after a hysterectomy, you won't be able to have more children.

We asked the women we interviewed if they had had a hysterectomy. Here is what they had to say about it:

> "This was tough. By the time I had the hysterectomy, I had two recurrences and had been dealing with GTN for 18 months. It was an emotional volcano for me. My doctor recommended a total hysterectomy (goodbye ovaries!). Knowing I wouldn't be able to have biological children, dealing with early menopause, feeling scared that the cells had spread by now (they were still contained), and feeling "defeated" by this illness as hard as I tried to "defeat it" [was tough]. After the surgery I was in a lot of pain, physically and emotionally. This was the hardest period of time for me since

all along I had hoped that I could "beat the odds" and have a child some day (through in-vitro or whatever). I had lived on hope, and now that hope was taken from me—although I knew intellectually that my life was given back to me, and that I could now start on the real road to recovery." (Diagnosed at 41 in 1999; treated in Memphis, TN, then Fort Lauderdale, FL.)

"The procedure was relatively easy. Post-surgical pain was bearable. I was up and walking on the third day. What was difficult for me was to make the final decision to have it done. You see I wanted to have another child, at the least." (Diagnosed at 36 in 1993; treated in Manila, Philippines, and Kuala Lumpur, Malaysia.)

The Different Types of Hysterectomy Procedures

- *Total Hysterectomy.* This involves the removal of the uterus and cervix through a horizontal midline incision just above the pubic bone (sometimes called a Pfannenstiel or bikini line incision). If your uterus is enlarged due to fibroids or from the GTN itself, then a vertical incision on the lower abdomen may be used instead. If you undergo this type of hysterectomy you'll no longer experience menstruation; however, you may continue to experience premenstrual signs (PMS) since the ovaries, which produce the hormones that cause PMS, may still be intact. You'll also no longer need to go in for an annual pap smear since your cervix will have been removed (a pap smear tests cervical cells).

- *Subtotal Hysterectomy.* This is the removal of the uterus without the removal of the cervix. Leaving the cervix intact has the advantage of reducing the chance of infection. Some women report a preference for this type of hysterectomy since it preserves more sexual response (for some women the cervix is implicated in orgasm). However, this factor is controversial and may be different for each woman. You'll no longer experience menstruation; however, you may continue to experience premenstrual signs (PMS) since the ovaries, which produce the hormones that cause PMS may still be intact. Since the cervix is intact you'll still have to go in for yearly pap smears to test for cervical cancer.

- *Hysterectomy with Bilateral Salpingo-Oophorectomy (BSO).* The BSO operation doesn't actually refer to a hysterectomy (removal of the uterus); it refers to the removal of the ovaries and fallopian tubes. It's included here because it's usually carried out at the same time as a total or subtotal hysterectomy. This operation is done to prevent ovarian cancer and ovarian cysts. If you have this operation you'll no longer experience menstruation, and you'll no longer experience premenstrual signs (PMS) since the ovaries, which produce the hormones that cause PMS, have been removed. In premenopausal women the sudden decrease in estrogen might cause menopausal symptoms. In general, removal of the ovaries is not recommended unless it's absolutely necessary (for example, there are metastasis on the ovaries). If you're premenopausal and your ovaries have been removed, you'll experience surgically-induced premature menopause.

- *Hysterectomy with Ovarian Conservation.* If a hysterectomy is performed before menopause and the ovaries are left intact, the ovaries will continue to produce hormones. You may continue to experience premenstrual signs (PMS) such as breast tenderness, bloating and irritability, though you'll no longer have a period (bleed) since the uterus has been removed. However, even with ovarian conservation, there may be a decrease in the amount of hormones produced since the blood supply to the ovaries may have been disturbed by the hysterectomy.

- *Radical Hysterectomy (Wertheims Hysterectomy).* This is an extensive hysterectomy wherein the uterus, ovaries, fallopian tubes, ligaments, surrounding tissues, pelvic lymph glands and upper third of the vagina are removed. In young women the doctor may decide not to remove the ovaries, or to transplant ovarian tissue to another part of the body for continued hormone production. This type of hysterectomy is usually only performed for cervical cancer, but might be performed if the GTN involves the tissue surrounding the uterus.

- *Vaginal hysterectomy.* This type of hysterectomy leaves no visible scar. The uterus is removed through the opening to the vagina rather than through a cut in the abdomen. However, this type of operation is usually not performed in the case of cancer, as the upper abdomen cannot be assessed for possible spread. The operation is easier to perform when a woman has undergone prior vaginal childbirth.

- *Laproscopic Hysterectomy.* In laproscopic hysterectomy a small cut is made into the abdomen, usually in the belly button. Carbon dioxide is then used to inflate the abdominal wall. A camera is inserted into the abdomen, and then several other small incisions are made in the lower abdomen to insert the instruments that will be used in surgery. The ligaments that attach the uterus to the abdominal cavity are severed and the vagina is opened to remove the uterus vaginally. Studies have shown that the laproscopic approach has a more rapid recovery, fewer complications, shorter hospitalization and less need for anesthetics. However, this technique is not available everywhere because it requires special equipment and a specially trained surgeon.

Adapted from the article by Hillary Walsgrove, "Hysterectomy." Nursing Standard 15(29): 47-55, April 4, 2001.

No matter what type of hysterectomy you receive, it's usually a very safe operation. Hysterectomy rarely causes serious, life-threatening complications. However, mild complications are common. Some studies suggest that about half of women who have a hysterectomy will have some form of mild complication, such as infection, hemorrhage, urinary problems, bowel problems, psychological problems or premature ovarian failure. Physical side effects may last up to a year after surgery; the most common of these is fatigue.

Psychological adjustment can be difficult if you've had a hysterectomy. You'll probably experience some anxiety about the surgery (most surgery patients experience anxiety before the operation). Informing yourself about what will happen during surgery is a good way to minimize this anxiety. Many women find that they have an altered self-image and a different view of their femininity after a hysterectomy. In our culture the womb is strongly associated with femininity, and losing your womb might make you feel un-sexy for a while (please see chapter 7 for more information on sex and sexual self-image after GTN treatment). Some women think their scar is ugly, while others look at as a sign of their bravery. If you think the appearance of a scar will bother you, you may be able to request a laparoscopic hysterectomy or vaginal hysterectomy.

Certain cultural beliefs may affect a woman's psychological adjustment to a hysterectomy. Some West Indians view menstruation as a cleansing act, which rids the body of impurities. After a hysterectomy, menstruation stops. This may cause the woman to feel impure. A hysterectomy can be devastating for some Muslim women, since in some Muslim countries, a woman's social role is dependent on her fertility. In Western societies, great emphasis and value is placed on youth. Women who experience early menopause as a result of their hysterectomy may feel that they're losing their youth.

There are numerous myths surrounding hysterectomy, which can cause groundless fears for the patient. You may have heard that a hysterectomy causes masculinization and the end of your sexual life. You may have heard that it causes weight gain or that you'll become unattractive. You may fear that your husband will reject you because of the hysterectomy. However, there's mounting evidence that shows that a hysterectomy may actually *improve* your sex life, especially if it was performed to help with a problem that was interfering with your sex life (such as the constant bleeding from GTN). Many women also welcome the fact that they no longer need to buy sanitary napkins and tampons.

When the doctors and nurses in the OR told me that they were going to do a hysterectomy on me, I was perfectly fine with it. I was shaking so badly I could hardly breathe, and was going in and out of consciousness because of the pain and loss of blood. All I could think of was "do something, *anything.*" After the operation, I was doped up on morphine—I didn't know which way was up! I kept seeing different pictures inside the picture that was hanging on the wall in front of me in my hospital room. I'd fall asleep in the middle of a sentence, then wake up and finish what I was saying as if nothing had happened! I must have been quite humorous! The reality of the operation didn't "hit" me until about a week after I got home. I was still in a lot of pain, and as a result we had a lot of family staying with us (clearly I gave them all a scare). I was so confused as to what actually happened, what they did, and so on.

Then came the thoughts of not being able to have more children. I was devastated. It felt like I had lost an actual baby. It felt like grief. Like I was a failure in a sense, that my body had failed me. We'd planned on having one more child, and it really bothered me that I'd been robbed of this option. It still does, although I've learned to deal with it, and have realized there's nothing I can do about it. Except to be happy that I don't have to go through any more periods! I'm still quite confused about how to feel at times, especially when I see a baby. I do know that I'm lucky to have my daughter and my stepson.

What to Expect When You Go Home After a Hysterectomy

For the first few weeks you may be tired and have little energy. You may have days when you feel in low spirits and cry for no apparent reason. These symptoms will probably pass. You may notice some discharge or bleeding from your vagina while the sutures heal. You can begin to move around, but you should begin with light exercise (such as walking around the house) when you first arrive home. Then you can gradually increase your activity as you regain some energy. You should avoid lifting or causing any strain on the abdominal and pelvic floor muscles. Approximately six weeks after the operation you can begin to exercise, swim and work again, if you feel up to it. Most women can also resume sexual intercourse after six weeks, although it's discouraged before this time in order to allow for adequate healing. Until then you can use mutual masturbation or holding and cuddling to express affection (see chapter 7 for more on sex during GTN treatment). You should also avoid sports and vigorous activities for about three months after the operation.

If you've had your ovaries removed, you may want to consider hormone replacement therapy (HRT). Talk to your doctor about whether this might be right for you. There are new drugs called "selective estrogen receptor modulators," which appear to help reduce the chance of developing osteoporosis and cardiovascular disease due to premature menopause. There are also natural alternatives to HRT. Some women eat foods that contain phytoestrogens (phytoestrogens are estrogens found in foods such as yams and soy products) to help with loss of estrogen. There are also homeopathic and herbal remedies, as well as reflexology, acupuncture and relaxation therapies, which some women find help with premature menopause.

Other Surgeries

You may need other surgeries if the cancer has spread to different parts of your body. Your doctor will be able to provide you with information regarding the type of surgery that will be used and how this surgery will be performed. Unfortunately we cannot comment on all the possible surgeries here, since the other surgeries used will be unique to you, depending on where you've had metastases.

The "chorio ladies" told us about their surgeries to remove metastasis:

"I had two brain surgeries to remove hemorrhages and metastasis. I don't remember [what it was like] and I don't remember [how it felt]. I don't remember [what I was thinking]." (Diagnosed at 31 in 1994; treated in Cleveland, OH.)

"[I had a] thoracotomy—surgical removal of lung tissue. It was a major surgery with post-surgical pain needing painkillers over several days. [At the time all I was thinking was] when will I go home?!" (Diagnosed at 36 in 1993, Treated in Manila, Philippines, and Kuala Lumpur, Malaysia.)

GTN TREATMENT PARTICULARS: CHEMOTHERAPY

Chemotherapy is the second most common form of GTN treatment. It's used to treat any abnormal placental cells that were left over after surgery. If the disease has spread to other locations that aren't easily reached by surgery, then chemotherapy will be used since it can travel throughout your body to work on even hard-to-reach cells. For information about the specific chemotherapy drugs that you are prescribed, please see the B.C. Cancer Agency Drug Manual or CancerBACUP Chemotherapy Drug Manual, listed in the resources at the back of this book.

What is Chemotherapy?

Chemotherapy refers simply to the treating of disease with drugs or medications. Many diseases are treated using drugs. However, chemotherapy is most often used in connection with cancer therapy. Chemotherapy treats the whole body rather than just a specific area. The drugs travel throughout your body's systems. In some cases a doctor will decide to use just one type of chemotherapy drug. This is called single-agent therapy. In other cases, or at a later date in the same case, a number of different drugs may be combined. This type of chemotherapy is called combination chemotherapy, or muti-agent therapy. If chemotherapy is given after surgery or after radiation therapy, it's called adjuvant chemotherapy. And if chemotherapy is given before surgery or before radiation therapy, it's called neoadjuvant chemotherapy.

The goal of chemotherapy is usually to produce a complete cure or achieve remission. The goal of neoadjuvant chemotherapy is sometimes to shrink the tumor to the extent that it's possible to use surgery or radiation therapy. When chemotherapy is given after surgery or radiation therapy, the goal is to destroy any abnormal cells that may have been missed in order to prevent the GTN from coming back.

I started my first regimen of combination chemotherapy on February 14, 2001. I was admitted into the hospital, and early the next day went in for my emergency hysterectomy. I was given my second dose of chemo after the surgery, which was planned before anyone knew I'd be having the operation. The doctors decided to resume the chemo regimen since I still had cancer cells in my lungs. So, every week I went in for a "short" treatment and a "long" treatment.

If you're undergoing chemotherapy treatment, it's very important that you inform your doctor of *all* the medications that you're taking *before* you start treatment. This includes birth control, vitamins, supplements, herbs, and nonprescription drugs (such as cold pills, laxatives, headache medicines etc.). This is so important it might even be a good idea to make a list of all the bottles in your medicine cabinet. You may find some that you've forgotten you occasionally reach for. Chemotherapy can interact with other drugs, which can then make the chemotherapy less effective—and can even be fatally dangerous to you. When undergoing chemo, I wasn't allowed to take anything with the drug Aspirin, or an abundant amount of Vitamin C (because Vitamin C interacts with the chemo by keeping the chemo in your body). Many physicians also recommend against non-steroidal medications (NSAIDS) such as ibuprofen, naprosyn, etc., as these can impair platelet function (the blood cells that allow you to form blood clots to stop bleeding).

How Does Chemotherapy Work?

Cancer cells divide far more often than normal cells. Chemotherapy exploits this fact and treats cancer by preventing or stopping cell division. Some chemotherapy drugs work by preventing the cancer cells from beginning the process of cell division. Other chemotherapy drugs attack cancer cells *while* they're dividing. Still others work by attacking all the cells in a tumor, whether they're in the process of dividing or not.

Chemotherapy is most destructive to cancer cells because they divide so often. However, normal body cells must also divide, because they have a limited life span and need to be replaced, or because they were damaged and need to be replaced.

Chemotherapy treats your whole body, and thus travels throughout your entire system. This means that some of your body's normal, non-cancerous cells will also be affected by chemotherapy. It's this effect on normal body cells that causes the side effects associated with chemotherapy.

Many people are frightened by the prospect of chemotherapy's side effects. Some patients find they have few side effects, and some even continue working, while others experience dramatic side effects and need to take time to recover. It's important to remember that, despite the side effects, the treatments are important since they greatly increase your chances of survival. Furthermore, once chemotherapy is finished, most of the side effects will disappear (see chapter 5 for more on side effects).

I wasn't sure what to expect when I first started treatment. I mean, I haven't actually known anyone personally who has had to go through cancer treatment. I didn't know if the side effects would hit me right then and there, as soon as the chemo was administered. I didn't know if or when my hair would fall out. I didn't know if the chemo would hurt, or if I'd puke all over the place when they put the "poison" into my body. I was also worried because I knew that sometimes treatment can make you helpless, and I was a very do-it-myself type of woman. I was scared that I wouldn't be able to take care of myself, let alone my family, and I was also scared to ask for help. I didn't know how to do it. I wanted to be there for my husband and kids, but some days it just wasn't possible.

The women we interviewed told us about their first experiences with chemotherapy:

> "I did not get nauseated from it, except [as an] inpatient, the first night. When I was doing chemo I was immune to calories! I understand it's because it jacks up your metabolism so high. Did a real number on my meds when I finished chemo though." (Diagnosed at 31 in 1994; treated in Cleveland, OH.)

> "Very odd. I kept waiting for the predicted side effects to take effect straight away—not realizing that they would build up with time." (Diagnosed at 30 in 1997; treated in Sheffield, UK.)

> "The very first chemo session went like a breeze." (Diagnosed at 36 in 1993; treated in Manila, Philippines, and Kuala Lumpur, Malaysia.)

"Within hours after the first treatment I became violently ill. I was allergic to various medications such as Compazine and there wasn't much they could give me for vomiting. I really thought I was going to die." (Diagnosed at 27 in 1973; treated in Southampton, NY, and New York City, NY.)

Is Chemotherapy Painful?

Chemotherapy itself rarely causes pain. If you're taking chemotherapy orally, it will be no different than swallowing any other pill or liquid. If your drugs are injected, it will feel the same as receiving any other vaccination or shot. When the drugs are given by IV, you'll feel a pin prick as the needle is inserted, but this is no more painful than donating blood. If you feel any burning or discomfort, you should be sure to tell your doctor or nurse.

I found that the actual administering of chemo wasn't painful most of the time. A couple of times, however, the chemo drug would irritate my veins and I would get a burning sensation in my arm, but that would go away with a heating pad. Once I had an allergic reaction to cisplatin (one of the chemo drugs), and they had to dope me up with Benadryl and a steroid, dexamethazone. My chest got really tight and I found it hard to breathe, then my face swelled up and I had a tingling sensation all over. It was quite scary. But, the Benadryl helped completely. From then on I wasn't allowed to get cisplatin without the Benadryl beforehand.

Here is what the women we interviewed had to say about pain and chemotherapy:

"It wasn't painful for me but would make me very weak for a couple of days after I received it." (Diagnosed at 24 in 2001; treated in New York City, NY.)

"I started having side effects after two doses of actinomycin-D. I felt more nauseous than before, and my hair started to thin out. The pains were in my stomach and uterus, probably where the tumor was lodged (my lower right side). EMA-CO was okay for the first couple treatments, then the cumulative effects got to me. [I became] very tired and nauseous, [and experienced] bone pain (combined with the (effects of the Neupogen® shots) and overall achiness. I wouldn't say it was painful, more like the pain from needles. Oh yes, and the mouth sores, now those were painful.

Awful!" Diagnosed at 41 in 1999; treated in Memphis, TN, then Fort Lauderdale, FL.)

"It was nauseating and energy-sapping." (Diagnosed at 36 in 1993; treated in Manila, Philippines, and Kuala Lumpur, Malaysia.)

My Experience with Chemotherapy Treatments

I had my first treatment while I was an inpatient at the hospital. There had been some confusion about whether or not I was going in overnight. By the time they straightened everything out, however, I had to be admitted. This was definitely one of the best mix-ups I could have had, since my body's cancerous cells reacted to the chemo in both good and bad ways. These type of cancer cells (choriocarcinoma cells) are known for being "bleeders." They develop and spread at an enormous rate—but are "killed off" quickly too. So the tumor ended up ripping a hole in my uterus while the cancer cells were being "killed," and I started bleeding internally, which required immediate attention. This was what resulted in my emergency hysterectomy. If I hadn't already been admitted at that time, I might not have made it to the hospital quick enough for them to "save" me.

Actually, come to think of it, I definitely would have died. Even the nurses assigned to me that day told me a few weeks later that they thought they were going to lose me—and that I scared the begeebers out of them! Some insurance companies won't pay for this kind of admission, but if it's possible you may want to ask to be admitted to the hospital, at least for the first course of chemotherapy. That way help will be close at hand if you experience any problems. If you can't be admitted it's important to have a way to contact your doctor immediately if any problematic bleeding should occur.

I received my chemotherapy treatments using an intravenous (IV). Getting an IV put in every time I went for chemo was okay when I first started. But after being on chemo for a long period of time, my veins began to shrink and "roll." The nurse had to then dig the needle into my arm until she hit the vein. This became very painful for me since my veins were so "used" and worn out. This also caused major bruising (especially if my blood counts were low due to the chemo). That said, an IV (or any needle for that matter) doesn't seem to bother me when I'm feeling at my best, but when I'm worn out or not feeling all that great, an IV is absolutely excruciating. So, after about seven months of chemo, I decided to get a port (i.e., "PORT-A-CATH").

This is a metal device that's surgically implanted into your chest area, and it has a tube that ends up close to your heart. It protects your veins from the chemo drugs, and is very painless when compared with the "poking" you get from a needle. An hour before chemo, I put a numbing gel on (e.g., "EMLA" cream), and when they inserted the needle I couldn't feel a thing! I'm kicking myself in the butt now that I didn't get this sooner.

There's another option that doesn't require surgery. It's called a peripherally inserted central catheter (PICC) line. Many places would rather put a PICC line through because it means one less surgery, and because it's easily done without booking an operating room. I weighed the pros and cons of both, and decided on the port, partly because I had a one year-old running around, and with the PICC line attached to my arm, I knew it would have been ripped out accidentally. You also can't get the PICC wet, which means no swimming or showering freely, and you also have to take extra care of the dressings. I decided I had enough to worry about, and didn't need the extra hassle of having to go in to change the dressing and so on. With the port, after you're finished chemo, the doctors recommend a time to go in and get it flushed (wherein they administer saline and a blood thinner called Heparin to make sure it doesn't clot up). This can be done more often, but you shouldn't go longer than two months in between flushings.

Since it can be pretty boring to sit with an IV in your arm, it's a good idea to come to the hospital with some activities or a book to keep you occupied. I found, when I first started chemo, that the all-day treatments seemed to last forever. I couldn't get up and walk around, and was confined to either a chair or a bed (which I had to request frequently). So, since Meredith and I were writing this book, I would bring in medical journals to read so that I could learn more about this type of cancer. I was also really lucky that my husband worked nights and that he was very supportive when it came to my going to the cancer center to get treatments. He would be there by my side almost the entire day. So, although he slept most of the time, I had someone to talk to and keep me company if I needed it. (Yep, I was mean and woke him up!) Once I started getting the Benadryl before every treatment, it would knock me right out, and I'd sleep until the treatment was over.

When I was first diagnosed, my oncologist estimated that my treatment would take about eight weeks. I was excited to hear that it would be so short. But I was also very skeptical. Needless to say, I received a little under a year and two months of straight chemo, with breaks here and there when I was admitted into the hospital or when my WBC count or hemoglobin were too low. I also had some tricky spots on my lungs that they had problems getting to. But that's just me. Other women go three months and are cured. It is weird, though, that *I knew* it would be a tough battle for me, and that it would take longer than they expected. I just wasn't expecting it to take quite so long. It scares me to this day, but I've realized that it's normal to think this way. If you end up having stubborn cancer cells, you just have to deal with it the best you can!

COMPLEMENTARY AND ALTERNATIVE THERAPIES

A therapy is called complementary when it's used in *addition* to conventional treatments. A therapy is called alternative when it's used *instead* of conventional treatments. Conventional treatments are those that are widely accepted and practiced by the mainstream medical community (a.k.a. the Western medical community). Complementary and alternative therapies are used in an attempt to prevent illness, reduce stress, prevent or reduce side effects and symptoms, or control and cure disease.

The use of complementary and alternative therapies is very widespread. Patients who choose to use complementary and alternative medicine report that the choice represents an attempt to gain greater control and decision-making power over their medical treatment. They believe that their conventional practitioner is truthful and has technical knowledge; however, they also value their complementary therapist(s) for providing emotional support and for listening.

Less is known about complementary and alternative therapies than conventional therapies. This is because, while a lot of anecdotal information about these therapies exists, very few of them have been submitted to rigorous scientific testing. However, scientific knowledge isn't the only form of knowledge. This is easy to forget in our modern era, where the words "scientifically proven" carry great force. Before the scientific method was invented, people still knew things. The difference that the scientific method brought about was the introduction of careful controls to eliminate bias. Often people see what they want to see, and science offers a way around this distortion. If you choose to use complementary and alternative medicines (CAMs) you still need to exercise caution, since most of the anecdotal evidence for herbal medicines comes from a time before chemotherapy. Even if a treatment may have helped in the past, it may be harmful in the present, due to its interactions with conventional treatment.

If you're considering using complementary and alternative therapies yourself, you should discuss this decision with your oncologist. Some of these therapies may interfere with your chemotherapy, or may be harmful when combined with the chemotherapy drugs. Your oncologist and your alternative practitioner should work together wherever possible. A good alternative therapist will welcome this opportunity for collaboration. Beware of any alternative therapist who's reluctant to consult with your oncologist. If your practitioner won't work with your cancer specialist, it's best to look for care someplace else.

When deciding whether to use complementary therapies you should ask questions of your alternative care practitioner, your oncologist and yourself. Take a look at the following examples:

What to Ask Your Alternative Therapist Before Beginning Treatment

- Ask your practitioner about his or her experience. You might want to inquire about credentials, practice experience, familiarity with your type of GTN, and names of other patients you might contact for reference.
- Ask about the risks and benefits of the treatment. Beware of any practitioner who says there are absolutely no risks or safety issues.
- Ask about side effects.
- Ask what results you can expect from the therapy. Beware of any practitioner who claims to have a "miracle cure" that treats any condition with guaranteed results.
- Ask how many treatments will be required before you see results. Beware of practitioners who won't tell you how long the treatments will take or when you can expect to see results.
- Ask how much each treatment costs and how much the therapist expects your whole course of treatments will cost. Beware of any therapist who won't give you an idea of how much your treatment will cost.
- Ask which herbs or substances will be used in your therapy. Make a written list and show this to your oncologist. Beware of any products that your oncologist cannot identify after doing a thorough search.

Also use caution if the product contains "secret" ingredients. Never use any therapy that requires getting shots of any kind without talking to your oncologist first.

- Ask whether there is research that shows how safe and effective the therapy is. If you aren't comfortable evaluating research (and even if you are) you should show these documents to your oncologist and ask him or her to evaluate them. S/he may be able to help you decide whether the therapy will be safe for you in combination with your particular treatment protocol.
- Ask whether your oncologist can call and consult with your alternative practitioner. Beware of any therapist who refuses to consult with your oncologist.

Adapted from The American Cancer Society's website "An Overview of Complementary and Alternative therapies" and The National Cancer Institute's website "Complementary and Alternative Medicine in Cancer Treatment: Questions and Answers."

Once you have answers to these questions from your complementary care practitioner, take a moment to evaluate them. If the claims are modest (remember, this is health and not "magic") and the practitioner is willing to work with your oncologist, this is the first sign that the complementary therapy may be right for you. When considering the answers to these questions, remember that "natural" doesn't mean "safe." There are plenty of natural products that are extremely harmful (just think of hemlock, a powerful poison).

So, just to recap:

- Avoid products that are likely to interfere with your conventional cancer treatment.
- Beware of dangerous or poisonous ingredients that may lead to adverse effects (use special caution if there are "secret" or hidden ingredients).
- Avoid any treatment that requires the excessive use of a particular herb or product. Use in moderation should be your motto.
- Beware of any treatment that involves exorbitant costs.
- Even some minor alternative treatments can cause problems with bleeding so confirm that everything is safe *before* you take it.

If you feel inclined to keep your complementary therapy secret from your oncologist, this is a red flag that something is wrong. And if your complementary practitioner suggested that you keep it secret, you should be suspicious of the practitioner and seek care elsewhere. A website called "quack-watch" (*www.quackwatch.org*) offers information about alternative therapies and practitioners. You may want to check this site for information on your treatment or therapist.

And if it's your conventional practitioner who's making you feel uncom-fortable about discussing your treatment decisions, it's time to look carefully at your doctor-patient relationship (see pages 75–79).

Vitamins and Minerals

Some vitamins (like vitamin C) actually need to be avoided during certain chemotherapy protocols. Some minerals and vitamins are easier to digest when they're found in foods rather than in pill or powder form. Since chemo-therapy and radiation therapy can affect your digestion anyway, it's better to get your nutrients from food than from a pill, since your body may be able to draw even less benefit from the pill than normal. Ask your doctor before taking any vitamin or mineral supplement.

For more information, the American Cancer Society has a good web-page devoted to alternative therapies: American Cancer Society "Comple-mentary and Alternative Therapies" (*www.cancer.org/docroot/ETO/ETO_5.asp?sitearea=ETO*).

CHAPTER 6

COPING WITH THE SIDE EFFECTS OF CHEMOTHERAPY

GTN AND CHEMOTHERAPY

All forms of GTN may be treated with chemotherapy. Some patients find this confusing because we have a strong association between chemotherapy and cancer. Patients with non-cancerous forms of GTN may wonder why they are treated with "cancer drugs" when they do not have cancer. However, chemotherapy is very effective in treating GTN in both its cancerous and non-cancerous forms. Chemotherapy has the ability to spread through almost all of the body's systems, allowing it to reach GTN cells that could not be reached by surgery alone. For this reason chemotherapy is sometimes prescribed for GTN, even when the GTN is non-cancerous.

This section of the book offers a comprehensive look at the side effects most commonly associated with chemotherapy. If this chapter looks long and daunting, take heart, each patient reacts to chemotherapy differently, and you may not experience all of the side effects listed here. In fact when we interviewed women with choriocarcinoma, we found that most of them had only experienced one or two of the side effects we listed. The purpose of this section is to let you know what to expect, so that you're not shocked or concerned if you notice these symptoms. You may even be pleasantly surprised to find that your reaction to chemotherapy is actually quite mild.

On the other hand, you may be one of the unlucky patients who react quite severely to chemotherapy. If this is the case, then the purpose of this chapter is to give you information on ways to deal with the side effects. This section should help you to understand what's happening to your body and why. It will also help you to communicate your side effects to your doctor, and to assess side effects that are normal (and can wait until your next doctor's visit to be discussed) as opposed to side effects that are serious and require immediate attention.

Many of the things we've suggested you do to help deal with the side effects of chemotherapy are actually quite enjoyable. One of the keys to avoiding side effects is to relax—take a load off and let your friends and family take care of you! You need and deserve the rest.

I think I was one of the unlucky ones, seeing as I had many of the side effects mentioned in this chapter. It was really tough, but it does get better and life, as they say, goes on. One of the hardest things for me was the way I felt on a day-to-day basis. I didn't feel like myself at all, and I hated that. But, I have very understanding family and friends who helped me along the way—even if it was to just leave me alone!

THE PHYSICAL SIDE EFFECTS OF CHEMOTHERAPY TREATMENTS

In chapter 5 we looked at how chemotherapy works. You may remember that chemotherapy attacks the rapidly dividing cancer cells by preventing them from replicating. We also mentioned that chemotherapy affects the whole body, and not just the cancer cells. The side effects of chemotherapy are a result of the effects these drugs have on the healthy cells of your body. For this reason the body systems that require constant repair are the same body systems that are most affected by side effects. Each person's reaction to chemotherapy is different. It depends on your overall health and which chemo drugs you're on, because some of the chemos out there are a piece of cake compared to others. Taxol, for example, is reputedly the worst for breast cancer patients, yet I found it the easiest.

LOW BLOOD COUNTS

Blood cells are produced in your bone marrow. The three main types of blood cells are white blood cells, platelets and red blood cells. Blood cells reproduce often, and so are affected by chemotherapy.

Your doctor will carefully monitor your blood cell count while you're receiving chemotherapy. Before your treatments you'll have your blood drawn, and these samples will be sent to a lab. Your doctor may prescribe medications to help you produce blood cells. Your doctor may also decide to postpone your treatment or adjust your dosage if your blood cell count is too low.

White Blood Cells

White blood cells are called leukocytes. There are several kinds of white blood cells, and all of them help to protect your body from infection. White blood cells are involved in you immune response to fight off germs. Since chemotherapy reduces your number of white blood cells, it also makes you more susceptible to disease and infection. Low white blood cell counts make it more difficult to fight off any infection that does arise. So, it's important to avoid getting an infection while you're undergoing chemotherapy. The best way to avoid infection is to wash your hands frequently. If possible, avoid large gatherings of people, and always avoid contact with people who are sick with colds, flu and other contagious diseases.

Recently a new drug called Neupogen® was developed to help replace blood cells. This drug is invaluable as it allows a chemo patient's treatment to continue at a regular interval (she no longer has to wait for her white blood cells to recover on their own). However, some patients find that Neupogen® has side effects that they can't tolerate, and these patients may prefer to wait it out. Now there are also longer acting-forms of treatment, such as Neulasta, that only require one shot. As always, you should discuss these options with your doctor.

I was asked to take Neupogen® the third time I went in for treatment. TJ was to give me shots, which I preferred taking in the leg, in between my treatments. After the first few days of getting this shot, I experienced major back pains. I couldn't sit or lie down without hurting really badly—so I had to pace. Then I'd get tired of pacing. I was such a wreck! I remember starting to bawl, and trying to tell my dad what the pain was like. It felt like a migraine, but in my lower back. There was a major throbbing that would increase whenever I sat down. After that, I switched doctors and my bloodwork was monitored every couple of days to see if and when I needed the shot. It turns out that I reacted amazingly well to the Neupogen® shot, and really didn't need as high a dose as my first doctor had prescribed.

I'm not usually scared of needles, but this one really scared me. When the Neupogen® goes in, it stings. And it makes sense that if your body is already worn out from chemo and you're not feeling all that great, that's when needles hurt the worst.

Tips to Help You Avoid Infection
- Wash your hands often. Wash them for at least 20 seconds (you can sing "Happy Birthday" to yourself twice, and that should be enough time). Also be sure to wash your hands before eating and after using the washroom.
- Avoid crowded places where you may come into contact with people who have contagious illnesses.

113

- Keep a bottle of hand sanitizer around and use it liberally!
- Don't tear the cuticles from your nails. This can cause cuts, which can then allow infection into your body. Your skin is a natural barrier to disease and infection. Try to keep it intact. Use an electric razor instead of a regular razor to prevent nicks. Also avoid squeezing pimples and blackheads. If you do get a cut or nick on your skin, wash the area with soap and water immediately.
- Use a soft toothbrush to prevent your gums from bleeding. Bleeding gums signal the presence of tiny cuts, which (as explained above) are openings into your body where infection can enter.
- Take a warm shower every day and pat your skin dry rather than rubbing it briskly.
- If your skin is dry or cracked use a lotion to promote healing. Ask your doctor or pharmacist to suggest a good brand (Eucerin, Aquaphor, and Bag Balm are excellent).
- After each bowel movement, clean your rectal area gently, but thoroughly. If you have hemorrhoids ask your doctor or nurse for advice.

How to Avoid Food-Borne Illness
- Wash your hands before and after preparing food (for at least 20 seconds).
- Wash all surfaces before preparing food (this includes knives and cutting boards). You may want to dedicate a special cutting board for meat, one for fish and another for raw vegetables.
- Wash all raw fruits and vegetables well. Scrub rough surfaces, such as the skin of melons and oranges, before cutting.
- Thaw meat in the refrigerator rather than on the counter.
- Cook meat and eggs thoroughly.
- Avoid raw shellfish.
- Use only pasteurized milk and cheese.
- Use only processed juices and ciders.
- Decant tomato juice if it comes in a can. Store it in a plastic or glass container instead.

Adapted from National Cancer Institute's webpage "Eating Hints For Cancer Patients," the Canadian Cancer Society's booklet "Chemotherapy and You" and the American Cancer Society's webpage "Understanding Chemotherapy."

Even if you take all of these precautions, it's still possible that you'll develop an infection. This isn't your fault. Viruses and bacteria have evolved to the extent that they can exploit any opportunity just to get inside the human body. That said, it's important to know what to look out for.

Common Signs of Infection

- White patches or a white coating in your mouth.
- A fever above 38°C (100.4°F) that lasts more than 2 to 3 hours. You should monitor your temperature, but you should *not* use Aspirin or other medications to reduce your fever unless advised to do so by your doctor or nurse.
- Sweating, especially at night.
- Diarrhea.
- A burning sensation when urinating.
- Severe cough or sore throat.

Adapted from the Canadian Cancer Society's booklet "Chemotherapy and You" and the American Cancer Society's webpage "Understanding Chemotherapy."

Platelets

Platelets are called thrombocytes. Platelets help your blood form clots in order to stop the bleeding if you're cut or bruised. When your platelet count is low, you may find that you bruise more easily. You may find that you bruise even from minor injuries that wouldn't have affected you at previously.

If your platelet count becomes too low you may need a platelet transfusion. (If you are a Jehovah's Witness you may want to discuss this with your religious advisor, since some congregations consider this type of transfusion acceptable, whereas other forms of transfusions are not.) If you notice that you're bruising easily or if you notice red spots under your skin, let your doctor know, as this may indicate low platelets. You should also let your doctor know if you experience unusual bleeding from your gums, nose, bladder, vagina or rectum.

When my platelets were low, I'd bruise very easily. If you cut yourself, you have to be extra cautious because your blood won't clot as quickly, if at all, depending on how low your count is. As one of the ladies on the Yahoo Choriocarcinoma Support site says: "If your platelets are low, you better not be shaving your legs or anything." I always got a chuckle out of that because I was hairless when she said that to me! I would get mouth sores, vaginal dryness and itch, and my hemorrhoids would act up. However, I'd only experience this when my platelets were low.

How to Avoid Problems When Your Platelet Count Is Low

- Do not take any over the counter pain medications (especially ASA, ibuprofen, naprosyn) since these may "thin" your blood. You can use plain Tylenol or acetaminophen.
- Do not floss your teeth. Use a cotton swab to clean your teeth rather than a toothbrush.
- Do not pick your nose. This can scratch the lining of your nose and cause bleeding. Use a tissue instead.
- Try to avoid getting constipated (see pages 129–130).
- Be extra careful to avoid burns, especially when cooking. Always use a hot pad to take things out of the oven.
- Avoid contact sports or other activities that may result in injury (swimming, walking and careful bike riding are okay).
- Be extra careful when using sharp tools, such as knives or saws. Always wear protective gloves when doing heavy work.
- Wear gardening gloves while tending your flowers to avoid being pricked by thorns.

Adapted from the Canadian Cancer Society's booklet "Chemotherapy and You" and the American Cancer Society's webpage "Understanding Chemotherapy."

Red Blood Cells

Red blood cells are called erythrocytes. Red blood cells carry hemoglobin, which in turn carries oxygen, to all of the parts of your body. This is essential, since your cells need oxygen to function. If your cells don't get enough oxygen, they won't do their jobs properly. This condition is called anemia.

Anemia causes you to feel extremely tired. So get plenty of rest and conserve your energy. When my hemoglobin was low, I was in dire need of a transfusion. You could just see it in my face—I looked like a walking ghost! My doctor would wait until it got down to a certain number before I could go in for a transfusion. I'd be so tired. I'd sleep most of the time and I'd some-

116

times have to crawl to the bathroom. My homecare nurse would come, and I couldn't even sit up for her to take my blood pressure, or get up the energy to talk to her (she was a chatty one—and no, I'm not complaining!).

After a while though, your body gets used to functioning with a lower than normal blood count. It's even possible to feel somewhat normal on the energy level front (I guess as normal as you can while you're on chemo) even when your counts aren't anywhere near the lowest "normal" number.

A low red blood cell count may also make you feel dizzy, chilly or short of breath. Move slowly to avoid getting dizzy. (Instead of jumping out of bed, sit up first. Wait a moment. Move to the edge of the bed. Wait a moment. Then stand up. Don't rush) If you're extremely anemic you may require a blood transfusion. Furthermore, there are new injection drugs (Procrit or Aranasp) that your doctor can prescribe along with iron to help your bone marrow produce more red blood cells to help combat anemia. If you feel tired or dizzy be sure to report it to your doctor, as this may signal a problem with your red blood cell count.

FATIGUE

Fatigue is characterized by a loss of energy or feelings of tiredness. Fatigue is the most commonly reported side effect of chemotherapy. Fatigue gradually increases over the course of therapy. The longer your treatments last, the more likely you are to experience fatigue. Between 82 and 96 percent of patients undergoing chemotherapy report fatigue. Fatigue affects your quality of life because it makes it more difficult to do the things you once enjoyed. Furthermore, studies have reported that when fatigue increases, a patient's experience of other side effects is often worse. It can be very tiring to be tired all the time!

Even though this is one of the most common side effects, it's one of the least studied. This is because it's difficult to measure a subjective quality like fatigue.

I experienced fatigue. It would frustrate me, because the house would be unorganized or messy and I'd want to clean up, but I couldn't muster the energy or the oomph to get off the couch, or out of bed. I'd try to go for a walk and I'd walk really slowly, stopping for a break every quarter block. My fatigue got a little better after I moved to Saskatchewan because I switched chemo protocols again (to the taxol), and getting all the EP-EMA out of my system was a big improvement. But I still didn't feel totally up to par, especially the night and next day after chemo—though I was certainly much better than with the EMA-CO and EP-EMA!

Fatigue is caused by a number of factors. First, red blood cell formation is affected by chemotherapy (see pages 116–117). Red blood cells carry hemoglobin, which carries oxygen, to all the cells in your body. When you don't get enough oxygen, your cells can't do their job. Usually this is caused by overexertion, and it's a sign that you need to rest. However in chemotherapy patients fatigue is chronic, and may not disappear after rest.

A decrease in white blood cells (see pages 112–115) is also thought to contribute to fatigue. Moreover, if you're experiencing diarrhea or vomiting, you may not be getting enough nutrients. This too contributes to fatigue.

Fatigue was one of the most reported side effects among the women we spoke with:

> "It interfered with everything I did. It seemed like my life was going in slow motion the whole time I was on chemo, and then for months after chemo stopped. It seemed the more I tried to do to make my energy level rise the more tired I was." (Diagnosed at 24 in 2001; treated in New York City, NY.)

> "The first day after chemo I'd be "flat" in bed. By the second day I'd be able to get up and about but I'd be sitting to rest very often. As the days went on I'd be able to do the usual light household chores during the day, but towards evening my energy level was almost drained out. I'd take afternoon naps. I'd take energy drinks during the day. I'd also stay away from heavy (high protein) dinners, which tended to make me very sleepy." (Diagnosed at 36 in 1993; treated in Manila, Philippines, and Kuala Lumpur, Malaysia.)

Tips for Dealing with Fatigue

- Give in to fatigue. If you're tired, rest. Don't try to push yourself.
- Take naps, but try to limit them to one hour.
- Remain as active as possible. Moderate exercise can help fatigue. But be realistic. Don't overexert yourself.
- Stick to a daily routine. Changes in routine require more energy from the body.
- Drink lots of fluids, as dehydration contributes to fatigue.

- Eat well, as a lack of nutrients contributes to fatigue.
- If your friends and family are looking for ways to help, you can suggest that they prepare some freezable meals for you and your family.
- If you don't have anyone to cook for you, prepare several meals (or larger portions of the meals you're already preparing) on days when you do feel well. You can freeze these and thaw them on days when you don't fell well.
- Buy healthy convenience foods that are easy to prepare. Many grocery stores offer a variety of prepared salads and main entrees in their deli section.
- Ask about a "Meals on Wheels" program in your area. Your doctor may know of one that would be helpful to you.
- Use grocery delivery services to keep your shelves stocked even when you don't have the energy to go out and do the shopping.
- Use time-saving appliances like your microwave and food processor.
- Keep ready-made healthy snacks in the refrigerator (carrot and celery sticks keep well when stored in water).
- Try easier or shorter versions of your favorite recipes.
- Identify and avoid environments or activities that increase fatigue.

Adapted from National Cancer Institute's webpage "Eating Hints For Cancer Patients," the Canadian Cancer Society's booklet "Chemotherapy and You" and the American Cancer Society's webpage "Understanding Chemotherapy."

PAIN

Pain is a common side effect of chemotherapy. Pain can be intense and localized, or it can be dull and pervasive. Pain can sometimes move around. Many patients worry about experiencing pain from chemotherapy; however, most pain can be controlled. Communication is important. You must let your doctor know what kinds of pain you are experiencing, so that he or she can properly treat it. Whatever you do, don't just "grin and bear it."

Some patients worry about taking pain medication because they've heard that these medications are addictive. However, addiction is rare when opioids are used for pain relief. Where this is the case, addiction occurs in only 1 in 10,000 patients.

The pain I remember most was what I called the after-chemo achiness. It felt like my whole body was bruised all over—like I was in a car accident. Whenever I moved or when anything touched me, I was in pain. I found Aleve helped me the best with that.

Here is what the women we interviewed had to say about pain:

> "Yes, I had a lot of extreme pain before the diagnosis. I experienced pain every once in awhile in my sides because of the tumors. They prescribed me oxycodone for it, but I didn't like taking it because it would make me very nauseous and tired." (Diagnosed at 24 in 2001; Treated in New York City, NY.)

> "Sometimes I had period-type cramps, which were more painful than usual." (Diagnosed at 30 in 1997; Treated in Sheffield, United Kingdom.)

> "Initially I did and it was difficult. Medication helped as well as good care from my caregiver." (Diagnosed at 41 in 2002; treated in Pensacola, FL.)

Tips for Managing Pain

- Check with your doctor before taking any pain medication (including Tylenol, Advil, Aspirin, Aleve or other over-the-counter medications). Some of these may interact with your chemotherapy drugs to dangerous ends.
- Don't try to "tough it out." Some patients worry that if they take pain medications too soon, there won't be a medicine strong enough to control their pain if it gets worse later on. In fact, it's best to treat your pain when it begins since this will make it easier for the doctors to control it later on. It's best to stay "on top" of your pain. Your body won't become immune to pain medications.
- Keep a pain diary, or enlist a family member to keep track of your pain for you. Write down the time of day that you experienced the pain, and then rate the intensity of the pain on a scale of 1 to 10. Also keep track of the things you did to make the pain better.
- Engage in enjoyable activities to take your mind off the pain (listen to music, get a back-rub, take a warm bath, read or watch TV).
- Consider acupuncture, which has long been reported to help with pain. It's important to let your acupuncturist know that you're

receiving chemotherapy so that he or she can take extra precautions to avoid infection. If your platelet counts are low it's best to avoid acupuncture until they've recovered.

- Try stimulating the skin near the site of pain with pressure, warmth or cold to help lessen the experience of pain. Some patients also enjoy vibration or menthol preparations. (However, it isn't a good idea to vibrate the treatment area if you're receiving radiation therapy.)

Adapted from the Canadian Cancer Society's booklet "Chemotherapy and You" and the American Cancer Society's webpage "Understanding Chemotherapy."

DIGESTIVE PROBLEMS

The digestive system takes a lot of abuse. Since we need to eat every day, a large amount of traffic moves through the digestive system. Moreover, our digestive juices are highly concentrated acids, which tend to wear down the lining of the digestive tract. For this reason the cells of the digestive tract require constant renewal. When chemotherapy prevents rapid cell division, side effects in the digestive tract are often noticed.

If you've been given a special diet by a nutritionist or dietitian you should try to stick to it. If not, the main recommendation for dealing with all digestive problems is to eat small meals throughout the day (rather than two or three large meals), drink plenty of water or juice and get exercise. These habits are good for the digestive system and should be adapted by everyone, even those who aren't undergoing cancer therapy. This may be the perfect time to increase both your health and that of your family!

Tips to Avoid Nausea and Digestive Problems

- Eat slowly and chew your food well. Digestion actually begins in the mouth. Your saliva helps to break foods down. If you chew well your stomach's job is easier.
- Give in to your cravings—even if you might normally deny yourself the food because it's fattening or unhealthy. It's better to eat something than to eat nothing. Just try to ensure that you make healthy choices as well.
- Rest after meals, as activity may slow digestion.
- Try to drink fluids when you're not eating. Drinking and eating at

the same time can make you feel overly full.

- Try to relax before eating. If you've been rushing around all day your digestion may be slowed down. Listen to relaxing music, have a calming talk with a loved one, anything that makes you feel relaxed.
- Wear loose clothing. Constrictive clothing can interfere with your comfort while you're eating.

Adapted from the Canadian Association of Nurses in Oncology booklet "Feeling Your Best," the National Cancer Institute's webpage "Eating Hints For Cancer Patients," the Canadian Cancer Society's booklet "Chemotherapy and You" and the American Cancer Society's webpage "Understanding Chemotherapy."

I found it really hard to keep up with the exercise as well as eating and drinking. It would get to the point where I'd be hungry, have a huge bowl of macaroni (I found this one of the easiest things to eat), have two or three bites, and be full. Or, it didn't taste as good as it looked (or as I remembered it tasting before chemo). Also, I couldn't drink water. It would make me vomit, or make me sick to my stomach for the rest of the day.

Nausea and Vomiting

We naturally avoid foods that make us nauseous or that make us vomit. Under normal circumstances this is a helpful reaction since it protects us from eating foods that have been contaminated or that are unsafe. During chemotherapy, however, this helpful reaction becomes a problem. It isn't the food that's making you feel ill, it's a side effect from treatment. Food aversion can become a problem when you begin to dislike foods that you once loved.

Nausea and vomiting occur when chemotherapy affects the fast-dividing cells of the gastrointestinal tract. Sometimes chemotherapy drugs also affect the part of the brain that controls vomiting. Fortunately, there have been recent advances in anti-nausea drugs (called antiemetics). Your doctor will probably prescribe a combination of antiemetic drugs since combinations have been found to be more effective than single drugs. But some people experience side effects from antiemetics. The most common side effects are sleepiness and dry mouth. Less common side effects include feeling jittery, restless and agitated, or having muscle spasms.

Some of the anti-nausea drugs would actually make me nauseous for a little while. It got to be really bad. My anti-nausea drugs weren't working anymore, and they had to give me a bunch of different ones. Some of them worked; others didn't. I was constantly nauseous, yet I only vomited a few times. My doctor and nurse really didn't think it was as bad as it actually was, until I saw them one day when I was in for bloodwork. Then they saw for themselves just how bad it really was.

Here is what the women we interviewed said about nausea and vomiting:

> "I never vomited during chemo but was very nauseous. I did vomit constantly, though, before they diagnosed me." (Diagnosed at 24 in 2001; treated in New York City, NY.)

> "[I vomited] very much. What helped [me] feel better? Antiemetics. [And I] kept ice in my mouth." (Diagnosed at 36 in 1993; treated in Manila, Philippines, and Kuala Lumpur, Malaysia.)

Tracking your pattern of nausea and vomiting may help you decide what action to take. Keep a record of your nausea and vomiting in which you answer the following questions:

1. When did it start?
2. How long does the vomiting last? Is it more than 24 hours? Is it more than 72 hours?
3. Is the nausea and vomiting interfering with my being able to eat and drink enough?
4. Is the nausea and vomiting preventing me from working and socializing?
5. What makes my nausea and vomiting worse?
6. What makes it better?

The answers to these questions may help you identify certain situations, foods or other triggers that make you feel ill. They'll also help you assess just how well your antiemetic medications are working.

Helpful Hints to Keep Nausea at Bay

- Avoid coffee and caffeinated tea since these foods dehydrate you. Drink juice or light sodas (flat ginger ale) instead. If you want a hot drink, try herbal tea or water with lemon.
- Try slow, deep breathing through your mouth if you feel ill.
- Try acupuncture. Some patients find that it's an effective means of controlling nausea.
- Try to find things to distract you from thinking about how ill you feel.
- If you wear dentures or partial dentures, leave these out on the day of treatment, since having objects in your mouth tends to promote vomiting.
- Open a window and get some fresh air.
- Keep track of how often and how much you're vomiting. Report this to your doctor since it may help him or her to decide how much medication you should be receiving.
- Rinse your mouth after vomiting with a mild salt solution. You can also try rinsing with a little lemon juice added to water.
- Place a cool washcloth over your eyes.
- Keep a bowl or bucket close by so that you won't have to sit by the toilet. Empty the bowl after vomiting and rinse it with cold water.
- Try to have someone give you a back rub to help you relax, and help lessen your nausea.
- Avoid eating in stuffy rooms that are too warm and lack air circulation.
- Avoid fatty fried foods, gravy and rich sauces (foods that are high in fat take longer to digest).
- Avoid fish and eggs (the odor may bother you).
- Avoid luncheon meats such as salami, pepperoni, bologna, etc., as well as bacon and sausages (these meats tend to be spicy, while processed meats are harder to digest).
- Avoid cooked brussel sprouts, cabbage, broccoli and cauliflower (these can be gassy).
- Avoid onions and garlic (the odor may make you feel ill).
- Avoid sour cream, cream cheese, cream and very sweet or rich desserts.

- Avoid large meals immediately before treatment. Opt instead for one of the drier foods listed below, and some juice.
- Avoid offensive odors when you're eating (e.g., perfume, smoke and food odors). If the smell of food makes you feel ill, try to stay away from the kitchen while meals are prepared (what a great excuse to let someone else pamper you!).
- Cook outdoors on a grill to eliminate offensive odors inside.
- Don't force yourself to eat when you're nauseated, as this may cause a permanent dislike of the food that you're trying to eat.
- Don't try to eat or drink until you have your vomiting under control. Then, try clear liquids such as bouillon.
- Eat foods at room temperature rather than when they're very hot or cold. Foods at room temperature have less of an aroma than hot foods. Hot and cold foods consumed at the same time may also worsen nausea.
- Take your anti-nausea medication one half to one full hour before eating so that it has time to take effect.
- Eat small meals throughout the day rather than three large meals. This will prevent you form feeling too full. It will also help to get some nutrition into your body in the event that you do vomit.
- If you experience nausea in the mornings, try eating dry toast or crackers *before* getting out of bed.
- Do try to eat something, as nausea is often worse on an empty stomach.
- After eating relax for at least half an hour in a seated position. If you feel you must lie down, keep your head elevated at least 12 inches above the level of your feet.
- If your stomach is really upset, try a clear liquid diet.
- Try drinking nutritional supplements through a straw. The straw can actually cut down on your ability to smell and taste the supplement.
- Try drinking chilled or frozen fluids. You can also freeze your drinks in ice cube trays or eat them as popsicles.
- Try dry foods such as toast, dry cereal, Melba toast, plain cookies and crackers. These foods can ease an upset stomach.
- Opt for fresh, frozen and canned fruits and vegetables, as they're easy on the tummy.

- Try eating cottage cheese, plain potatoes, pretzels and popcorn.
- Consider skinless broiled or baked chicken, or chicken soup broth.
- Try eating popsicles, Jell-O, sherbet or angel food cake for dessert.
- Use boiling bags to cut down on odors from cooking.
- Use the kitchen fan to help disperse odors from cooking.
- Call your doctor or nurse if your vomiting lasts for more than 24 hours, and doesn't seem to be getting better.
- Call your doctor or nurse if your vomiting is preventing you from swallowing pills or keeping your medication down.
- Let your doctor know if you are experiencing side effects from the antiemetics.

Adapted from the Canadian Association of Nurses in Oncology booklet "Feeling Your Best," the National Cancer Institute's webpage "Eating Hints For Cancer Patients," the Canadian Cancer Society's booklet "Chemotherapy and You" and the American Cancer Society's webpage "Understanding Chemotherapy."

Some people also experience nausea when they even *think* of having chemotherapy treatment (this affects about 25 percent of chemotherapy patients, and is called anticipatory nausea). It's caused by anxiety and the expectation of becoming sick. Many patients find that the sights, smells and environment of the treatment center elicit anticipatory nausea. This is a psychological problem, although the result can be a real physical reaction. The most important factor in developing anticipatory nausea seems to be a consistent experience of nausea and vomiting after treatment. Unfortunately, antiemetic (anti-nausea) drugs don't seem to work to control anticipatory nausea, though they may help to prevent nausea in the first place (so that you don't develop anticipatory nausea). They may also help you to relax and focus on things other than your treatment. Distract yourself, with any activity you find enjoyable.

My stomach would start to churn when we were driving to the hospital in the morning, but once we got there, I'd be fine. (I'm getting the churning tummy even thinking about the drive right now!) Just interacting and talking with the people who worked there and who I saw at least once a week calmed me down.

Helpful hints for Controlling Anticipatory Nausea

- Your doctor may have you take your medications in a scheduled manner for the first days after chemotherapy to prevent nausea from developing. Make sure you discuss this option.
- Take your antiemetic medications a few hours before your treatment begins. This may ease the fear of nausea.
- Try to relax before your treatments. Lying down or meditating may help some patients.
- Place a cool washcloth over your eyes when your treatment begins. This can help calm you down.
- Have a conversation with a friend or loved one—about something other than your cancer treatment. This can help take your mind off things.

Adapted from the Canadian Association of Nurses in Oncology booklet "Feeling Your Best," the National Cancer Institute's webpage "Eating Hints For Cancer Patients," the Canadian Cancer Society's booklet "Chemotherapy and You" and the American Cancer Society's webpage "Understanding Chemotherapy."

Diarrhea

Diarrhea, like nausea, is caused when chemotherapy drugs affect the cells that line the intestines. Some diarrhea is nothing to worry about, but do let your doctor know that you've experienced diarrhea at your next appointment, since there are many drugs that help control it. And, if you have diarrhea that continues for more than 24 hours or involves severe cramping or pain, call your doctor immediately. Diarrhea causes a loss of fluids and electrolytes, so it's very important to drink lots of water if you're experiencing this symptom.

I experienced diarrhea with its corresponding tummy grumbling, cramps, and so on. It usually happened the day after chemo, and it went from one extreme to the other. It was especially bad right after I had my hysterectomy, being on stool softeners and all. I could never get it all figured out, because once I'd finished taking the stool softeners, I still had the diarrhea! (It wouldn't last as long though.)

Some Hints to Help You Deal with Diarrhea

- Try grating an apple and allowing it to sit out until it's brown. The oxidized pectin (fruit sugar exposed to the air) is the same as the ingredients found in many commercial anti-diarrhea medications.
- A decoction prepared from pomegranate skin may help with diarrhea. To prepare the decoction, take 50 g of fresh pomegranate skin. Soak it in 800 ml of water for one hour. Boil until a quarter of the volume remains (200 ml). Store this mixture in a clean, dry bottle. A couple of tablespoons can be taken several times a day. You may also add half a teaspoon of honey to the decoction.
- Another helpful remedy is a sugar and salt solution. Mix one teaspoon of sugar and half a teaspoon of common salt in a cup of water. Small doses of this mixture (around a quarter cup) can be given whenever you want a drink. This helps to replace lost electrolytes.
- A paste made of sesame seeds (1 teaspoon) and a few tablespoons of goat's milk is beneficial.
- Drink plenty of fluids to replace those that have been lost through diarrhea. It's best to drink liquids at room temperature rather than when they're very hot or very cold.
- Avoid dairy foods, which may irritate your bowels. If you love milk-based foods try switching to lactose-reduced milk, yogurt or buttermilk.
- Avoid fatty, fried foods, rich sauces, caffeine, alcohol, chocolate, and tobacco products.
- Avoid gassy foods (onions, peas, beans, cabbage, broccoli, cauliflower, brussel sprouts, spicy foods, beer and carbonated beverages). Chewing gum may also make you feel gassy.
- Avoid raw fruits, vegetables and any high-fiber foods (whole grain breads, cereal, brown rice, nuts and seeds) if you feel diarrhea coming on.
- Try removing the skins, seeds and membranes from fruits and vegetables. Some people claim this makes them easier to digest. Canned or well-cooked fruits and vegetables may also be easier to digest.
- Eat smaller meals throughout the day, rather than three larger meals.
- Limit your activities after a meal to give your body time to digest your food.

128

- Limit your intake of foods that contain caffeine, such as coffee, tea and cola beverages.
- Limit your consumption of dried fruits, berries, rhubarb, legumes (e.g., lentils, kidney beans, lima beans), peas, corn, broccoli, spinach and nuts. They make diarrhea worse for some people.
- Drink only liquids if you feel diarrhea starting (clear broth, juice, clear water, popsicles, weak tea, or rice water—made by boiling rice in water and draining off the water before it is absorbed).
- When you feel like you can eat solids again, start with small amounts of foods that don't irritate the bowel, such as chicken, fish, eggs, white bread, canned vegetables, bananas, applesauce and smooth peanut butter.

Adapted from the National Cancer Institute's webpage "Eating Hints For Cancer Patients," the Canadian Cancer Society's booklet "Chemotherapy and You" and the American Cancer Society's webpage "Understanding Chemotherapy."

Constipation

Chemotherapy drugs can also cause constipation, as can the medications you've been given to control pain. Many opioids cause constipation, yet these are the most effective pain-control agents we have. If you haven't had a bowel movement for more than a day or two, you may need a laxative. You should consult with your doctor.

I'd get over diarrhea and it would turn into constipation. It hurt so badly. I also had hemorrhoids, which made things worse. Sitting on the toilet, popping blood vessels in my head trying to get it out so that my tummy would feel better, and wanting to find something to cut it out right then and there! What a horrible thing to consider now, but that's what I was thinking then. Afterwards, it would burn so badly (nothing helped with that) and I just felt like sitting in cold bath water to cool it off. I took stool softeners, which didn't really help with the constipated part—they just made me have diarrhea afterwards.

Constipation isn't life-threatening, but it's important that you address it, because untreated constipation can lead to a condition called fecal impaction. Fecal impaction is a condition characterized by an accumulation of feces in the bowel, and it can be fatal.

Helpful Hints for Dealing with Constipation
- Drink plenty of fluids (about 8 to 10 cups a day) to keep your stool soft.
- Drink a glass of warm milk before going to bed. This helps promote easy evacuation in the morning. In case of severe constipation, mix two teaspoons of castor oil into the milk.
- Drink one liter of warm water and walk around for a few minutes immediately after waking up in the morning. Remaining active helps to ease constipation.
- Drink lemon juice mixed with warm water two to three times a day to help ease constipation.
- Try taking one or two teaspoons of aloe gel twice a day.
- Get some exercise, including abdominal exercises.
- Find a private bathroom where you feel comfortable. Embarrassment about going to the bathroom increases constipation.
- Drink prune juice, or eat stewed prunes.
- Include high-fiber foods in your diet (bran, raw fruits, dried fruits such as prunes, raisins and apricots, raw vegetables, whole grain breads, cereals, and nuts). And remember that it's important to drink fluids such as water and juice when you eat fiber, otherwise it may actually make the constipation worse.

Adapted from the National Cancer Institute's webpage "Eating Hints For Cancer Patients," the Canadian Cancer Society's booklet "Chemotherapy and You" and the American Cancer Society's webpage "Understanding Chemotherapy."

Loss of Appetite

Loss of appetite is common in chemotherapy patients. If you don't feel hungry, or you don't feel like eating, it can be very difficult to motivate yourself to prepare a meal. This is especially true for patients who are also experiencing fatigue. However, since nutrition is essential to a good recovery from chemotherapy, you should try to eat—even if you feel that you're forcing yourself some of the time.

Tips to Help with Loss of Appetite

- Get plenty of rest.
- Take a walk before meals.
- Eat when you're hungry, rather than waiting for mealtimes. Eat small meals throughout the day to make up for your reduced appetite.
- Chew your food thoroughly. Since digestion starts in the mouth, this will help prevent you from feeling full prematurely.
- Try to avoid drinking fluids when you're eating. Drinking and eating at the same time can also make you feel full prematurely. Take liquids one-half to one full hour before your meals. If you need to drink to help you swallow, take only small sips. Drink after mealtimes rather than during your meal.
- Make your meals pleasurable. Use soft light, music or flowers—whatever makes you feel good.
- Use different colored foods and garnishes to make your meals more visually appealing.
- Ask your doctor or nurse if you can have a glass of wine or beer with your meal. This may increase your appetite (and give you something to look forward to!)
- Ask about a "Meals on Wheels" program in your community.
- Take advantage of time-saving appliances like your microwave and food processor.
- Make an effort to eat regularly, even if it's only a few mouthfuls at a time.
- Take medications with a nutritional supplement instead of with water (unless the medication needs to be taken on an empty stomach).
- Use meal replacements when you find it really hard to eat.
- Make every mouthful count! Don't fill up on low-calorie foods and beverages (coffee, tea and "diet" products).
- Try eating before bed.
- Take smaller portions so that you have the satisfaction of finishing a meal. You can always go back for more.
- Keep ready-to-eat snacks and food on hand (cheese and crackers, dried fruits, nuts, milkshakes, yogurt, pastries and baked goods, frozen dinner, frozen waffles or pancakes, cereals and puddings).

List on previous page adapted from the National Cancer Institute's webpage "Eating Hints For Cancer Patients," the Canadian Cancer Society's booklet "Chemotherapy and You" and the American Cancer Society's webpage "Understanding Chemotherapy."

MOUTH AND THROAT PROBLEMS

Chemotherapy can decrease the amount of saliva you produce. This therapy can also cause sores to form in your mouth and throat. When your mouth and throat are dry, eating can be painful and difficult. This situation puts patients at risk for malnutrition. If you're already having digestive difficulties once you've gotten the food inside you, pain during eating is only likely to aggravate the problem.

Some of the women we spoke with reported that they experienced a change in the flavor of their mouth Here's how one woman described it:

> "I experienced something [I would describe as] metallic mouth. Lemon drops helped." (Diagnosed at 41 in 1999; treated in Memphis, TN, then Fort Lauderdale, FL.)

Dryness of the Mouth and Throat

This is a very common side effect of chemotherapy. Unless it interferes with your eating, it usually isn't dangerous. If you experience severe dryness your doctor can prescribe artificial saliva.

I experienced dry mouth quite often. I'd try to chew gum, but the taste would be overpowering or gross, and would make my stomach upset. Drinking water would help a little, but that would also make me sick. I basically just stuck it out and it got better a few days after each chemo treatment.

One of the women we interviewed mentioned having problems with dry mouth as well:

> "My mouth became very dry and so did my throat. My tongue swelled up so bad that I had ridges on my tongue where the spaces were in my teeth. I also had sores in my mouth. All this made it very hard to eat. As a matter of fact, I couldn't eat for days. The dietician at Sloan Kettering came to see me and we discussed the problem as best we could because I had trouble speaking. After that she sent me up milkshakes. That way at least I was getting some nourishment." (Diagnosed at 27 in 1973; treated in Southampton, NY, and New York City, NY.)

Some Helpful Hints to Prevent or Combat Dry Mouth

- Drink lots of fluids, especially while you eat, to make swallowing easier.
- Suck on ice chips.
- Suck on sugarless candy or chew sugarless gum.
- Avoid alcohol and tobacco, which may aggravate the dryness.
- Process your foods in a blender and add some liquid.
- Avoid foods that stick to the roof of your mouth.
- Take small bites and chew thoroughly
- Try eating cottage cheese and yogurt, mashed potatoes (with butter), macaroni and cheese, and other noodles.
- Try eating guacamole that you prepare at home (so that it isn't spicy).
- Choose foods that are easy to chew and swallow.
- Opt for custards, puddings and gelatins, which are easy on the mouth.
- Cook foods until they're soft.
- If swallowing is difficult, try tilting your head back or moving it forward to help.
- Rinse your mouth before eating. You can use a solution of baking soda and water to rinse your mouth (1 tsp of baking soda to 2 cups of water, mixed well).
- If your mouth is very painful, eat soft, unseasoned foods such as eggs, pancakes, French toast, pasta and oatmeal.
- Cook or simmer your food in liquids, and make more stews.
- Eat moist foods such as fruit and ice cream.
- Eat and drink frequently throughout the day. Try eating every two hours and sipping drinks throughout the day.
- Moisten dry foods with butter, margarine, gravy, broth and sauces.
- Dip your food into your drink. Who doesn't enjoy a cookie dipped in milk?
- Put foods into the blender to make them smooth and easy to swallow.
- Eat soft, cold foods (ice cream, pudding, watermelon, baby food and Jell-O).
- Ask about anesthetic lozenges or sprays that can numb your mouth and throat long enough for you to eat.
- Use artificial saliva.

List on previous page adapted from the National Cancer Institute's webpage "Eating Hints For Cancer Patients," the Canadian Cancer Society's booklet "Chemotherapy and You" and the American Cancer Society's webpage "Understanding Chemotherapy."

Mouth Sores (Stomatitis)

The cells that line the mouth divide frequently. This is why the mouth heals so quickly! However, when chemotherapy drugs are interfering with cell division some patients develop sores in the mouth. This is called stomatitis. You should let your doctor know if you experience this side effect since it can sometimes (but not always) indicate a serious problem. Furthermore, your doctor may be able to prescribe a medication to numb the area.

I was lucky enough to not experience too many mouth sores. I got a few, and the few I got hurt really badly. I'd rinse and gargle with a baking soda and warm water mixture, and they'd be gone within the next couple of days. Eating was really tough, especially foods that required a lot of chewing, or a really wide-open mouth, or those that were salty or spicy.

Here is what the women we spoke with had to say about mouth sores:

"I only had them once but they were very bad. I was put in the hospital and put on morphine for the pain. My whole mouth was a sore and I couldn't eat for two weeks. The entire first layer [of skin] peeled off before a new layer grew in." (Diagnosed at 24 in 2001; treated in New York City, NY.)

"I took warm Chinese tea as substitute for drinking water. I did this when I was back home after treatment. It greatly helped stave off any mouth sore that was threatening to break out. If it did manage to break out, it wasn't as painful." (Diagnosed at 36 in 1993; treated in Manila, Philippines, and Kuala Lumpur, Malaysia.)

Hints to Help You Cope with Mouth Sores

- Avoid juices with a high acid content (tomato juice, orange juice, grapefruit juice).
- Avoid salt and spicy foods if they sting your mouth.
- Opt for foods that don't sting (apricot nectar, pear nectar, squash, beans, and peas).
- Keep your mouth and gums clean using a soft toothbrush or cotton swab. A clean mouth helps prevent infection.

Adapted from the National Cancer Institute's webpage "Eating Hints For Cancer Patients," the Canadian Cancer Society's booklet "Chemotherapy and You" and the American Cancer Society's webpage "Understanding Chemotherapy."

Some Mouth Care Techniques to Prevent Infection

Since your mouth is extra sensitive during chemotherapy, and especially susceptible to infection, it's important that you take special care of it.

- Brush your teeth after every meal and before bed. Use a soft toothbrush (the type made for babies is best) and a gentle touch. Clean often rather than vigorously since brushing too hard can damage the tissues in your mouth.
- Rinse your mouth with a solution consisting of 1 teaspoon salt or baking soda combined with 2 cups warm water. Don't use commercial mouthwash since it often contains alcohol, which can dry out the tissues of your mouth.
- Ask whether it's a good idea to floss. Most of the time it is a good idea to floss daily, but it may not be recommended while you're undergoing chemotherapy.
- If toothpaste makes your mouth sting, use baking soda applied with a Q-tip.
- Avoid sugary snacks that cause tooth decay.
- Use lip balm to keep your lips moistened.
- Remove your dentures to give your gums a rest.
- Let your dentist know that you're receiving chemotherapy before any dental appointments. Your dentist *must* consult with your doctor since chemotherapy makes you more susceptible to infection, and your dentist may need to take extra precautions.
- If you do develop mouth sores, your physician can prescribe a mouth rinse that combines several liquid drugs (Benadryl, Mylanta, Carafate and lidocaine), which help with inflammation and also ease the pain.

Adapted from the National Cancer Institute's webpage "Eating Hints For Cancer Patients," the Canadian Cancer Society's booklet "Chemotherapy and You" and the American Cancer Society's webpage "Understanding Chemotherapy."

Changes in Taste and Smell

Anybody who's taken a bite of food expecting it to be one thing and then finding out it's something else, knows what an unpleasant experience this is. When you're prepared for one flavor but experience another you often find the flavor you weren't expecting unappealing—even if you would have enjoyed it had you not been thinking of the first flavor. Chemotherapy may change the way that your taste buds function, which changes the way that food tastes. Some chemotherapy patients report that they can taste the drugs used in their chemotherapy *after* their treatments, which also affects the taste of their food. This means that chemotherapy patients are more likely to encounter a situation where they expect one taste yet experience another taste. You may find you no longer enjoy your favorite foods. You may also find that food you once found disgusting is now quite delicious. Some cancer patients report that they changed the staple foods in their diet throughout the course of their treatment for exactly this reason.

Tips to Help You Deal with Taste Changes

- Try marinating red meat if it tastes bitter. Try using soy sauce, fruit juice or wine vinegar. Some people find that cold meat tastes better than warm meat.
- Use plastic cutlery instead of metal cutlery if you find that food tastes metallic.
- Rinse your mouth often with baking soda and water (1 teaspoon baking soda mixed with 2 cups water). Also rinse your mouth before eating.
- Eat food at room temperature or food that's slightly cool rather than very hot.
- If red meat tastes bitter try eating poultry, fish, eggs, tofu or cheese as an alternative source of protein.
- Use extra seasonings such as oregano, basil or rosemary.
- Put a slice of real lemon in your water to stimulate saliva and taste (but do avoid artificial lemon).
- Try new foods only when you're feeling well.
- Choose foods that look appealing to you. This may compensate for lack of taste or smell.
- Opt for tart foods, which may help to overcome the metallic taste.

Examples are oranges, lemonade, cranberry juice, pickles, lemon custard or pudding.

- Use bacon, ham or onions to add flavor to vegetables.
- Avoid adding salt to spicy foods, since it will make them taste even hotter.
- For foods that taste too salty, add some sugar.
- For foods that taste too sweet, add a little salt.

Adapted from the National Cancer Institute's webpage "Eating Hints For Cancer Patients," the Canadian Cancer Society's booklet "Chemotherapy and You" and the American Cancer Society's webpage "Understanding Chemotherapy."

SKIN PROBLEMS

Chemotherapy can affect the way your skin regenerates. This sometimes leads to pruritus (itching), red, dry and peeling skin. Chemotherapy can also cause acne. And Methotrexate causes your skin to be extra-sensitive to the sun. It's important therefore to wear a good sunblock, stay in the shade whenever possible, and wear a wide-brimmed hat and protective clothing. Some chemotherapy drugs, such as actinomycin-D, can damage tissues if they leak out of the vein. If you experience burning, redness or pain near the injection site, let your doctor know immediately. If you develop a severe rash (especially if combined with difficulty breathing) you should go to an emergency room and contact your doctor immediately. This might indicate that you're having an allergic reaction. Most of these skin reactions will disappear within a few weeks of finishing radiation therapy or chemotherapy.

My skin was very dry and scaly. It would really bother me. Other than that the only problem I had was a sunburn caution with one of the chemo drugs I was taking, so I couldn't really be out in the sun at all without major protection. So, I went and bought a SPF 70. There was no way I was getting a tan, let alone a burn, with that puppy on!

Most of the women we spoke with did not report skin problems. Here are a couple who did:

> "My skin felt dry and flaky, grayish. I used a nice moisturizer to keep it as supple as possible, but it never looked very good!" (Diagnosed at 41 in 1999; treated in Memphis, TN, then Fort Lauderdale, FL.)

"My skin peeled off my body in various places. It started under my arms [then] my crotch, my behind. I thought it was the soap I was using. It took me a while to realize it was the chemo drugs." (Diagnosed at 27 in 1973; treated in Southampton, NY, and New York City, NY.)

Helpful Hints for Skin Problems

- Use cornstarch instead of commercial powders (which may contain perfumes and other irritants) to treat itchy skin. This is for chemotherapy patients only. If you're receiving radiation therapy, check with your doctor first.
- Use a humidifier to maintain a moist environment. Keep the house at a moderate temperature, because heat lowers humidity.
- Avoid using ointments (Vaseline or mineral oil). Ask your doctor about creams and lotions to help with dry skin.
- Don't scratch! As mentioned on pages 112–115, chemotherapy makes you prone to infection. Scratching can cause tears in the skin, which reduce the skin's ability to provide a barrier to infection. Instead of scratching try placing a cool washcloth or ice on the itchy areas. Some patients find that applying pressure to these areas helps alleviate the desire to scratch. If you're receiving radiation therapy you still can't scratch; however, you also can't put anything very hot or very cold on your treatment area.
- Avoid bathing in hot water (use water at a very mild temperature instead). Avoid bathing frequently or bathing longer than 30 minutes. Avoid using soaps with perfumes or detergents. Avoid adding bubble bath or bath oil to your tub. Instead, use mild soaps made for sensitive skin. Add a colloidal oatmeal treatment to your bath. Finally, if you're receiving radiation therapy, be sure to avoid washing the marks off your body.
- Avoid tight restrictive clothing. Avoid clothing made of wool, synthetics or harsh fibers. Instead, wear cotton or flannel. Avoid clothing and bed sheets laundered with detergent. Wash clothing and sheets with a mild soap designed for infant clothing (e.g., Dreft) or use a detergent that contains no perfumes (e.g., Tide Free). If you're receiving radiation therapy, choose clothes that can be thrown away

if they become stained by the ink marks on your skin.

- Avoid underarm and genital deodorants.
- Try using an oral antihistamine to combat itching.
- Ask your doctor about topical corticosteroids (unless you're undergoing radiation therapy).
- If you experience acne, keep your skin clean using mild soap, then use over-the-counter medications to treat the acne.
- Try to avoid prolonged exposure to the sun. If you're not receiving radiation therapy, wear a sunscreen with *at least* SPF 15 (you should do this anyway). You can also use zinc oxide, which completely blocks out the sun (it comes in fun colors as well!). Radiation therapy patients should avoid using any creams and lotions on the skin.
- Wear protective clothing (sheer materials can keep you protected *and* keep you cool!).

Adapted from the Canadian Cancer Society's booklet "Chemotherapy and You" and the American Cancer Society's webpage "Understanding Chemotherapy."

HAIR LOSS

Hair loss is probably the side effect most commonly associated with chemo-therapy. It can also be one of the most difficult effects to deal with since it's so visible, even to strangers. However, not all patients experience hair loss. It's impossible to predict how your hair will be affected by chemotherapy. However, no matter how extensive your hair loss, it will only be temporary. Your hair will grow back once your chemotherapy treatments are finished. Some chemotherapy patients even find that their hair begins to grow back before their treatments are finished.

Hair is another type of cell that reproduces constantly. Your hair is always growing, which requires the development of new cells. Chemotherapy causes the cells of the hair follicles to break off near the scalp. This can cause your hair to be reduced to only a half centimeter or less. On the positive side, it affects all the hair on your body, so you may not need to worry about shaving for a while!

Hair loss may begin almost as soon as you begin your treatments, or it may begin gradually, as your treatments progress. You may begin to notice that you're losing more hair in the shower or bath. There may be hair left on your pillow when you wake up. Or you may notice that there's more hair left in your brush. This may be the extent of your hair loss, resulting in thinner hair, or it may continue until you're bald.

It took a little while for me to lose all of my hair. I shaved it off before it all fell out because I wanted to get used to the feel and look of myself without hair, and because I was getting annoyed about having to change my pillow-case every morning (my hair would come out in clumps). I chose not to wear a wig (they're itchy and uncomfortable) and mainly wore bandannas. (In the winter, though, you really realize how cold it is when you don't have hair!) I found a toque that had long little braids attached to it. When I was wearing it, no one could tell I was really bald! It was great for those days when we were out in public and I didn't feel like having to deal with all the "looks" from people. Actually, in the winter, some people wear a toque to bed to keep their head warm. I just got used to covering my head with the blanket. One thing I told people was that I always wanted to see what I looked like bald, but I was too big of a chicken to do it before. Now I know!

Some patients get very depressed about losing their hair. Many women feel that their beauty is strongly linked to their hair. Other women look at this as an opportunity to experiment with hairstyles that they wouldn't normally try. I had days when I felt ugly and wished I had hair again. What really bothered me was when my eyelashes and eyebrows started falling out. They thinned out with the first two protocols, and in the last protocol I lost them completely. It was a huge shock to me, and I missed having them. They seemed to have added color (even though I was really pale) and definition to my face. But I got over it. And they grew back again, however slowly!

Hair loss was a very commonly reported side effect in our survey:

> "Yes and it made me feel brave and courageous. People were very polite. Never had anyone be rude." (Diagnosed at 41 in 2002; treated in Pensacola, FL.)

> "Yes, all of it the first time, none the second. Was nice; baldness is great. I discovered that I look good bald! I could see all of the scars on my head from the brain surgery! People were nicer. My neighbors who'd never liked us have been nicer to us to this day! [What helped the most was] a hat a friend gave me that said 'No Hair Day' on it!" (Diagnosed at 31 in 1994; treated in Cleveland, OH.)

"Yes, I lost most of my hair by the time I had my third chemo treatment. I had my husband shave it off when it got too thin. I'm not a vain person but it was probably more upsetting to me then the actual cancer. I know that sounds weird but it's the truth." (Diagnosed at 24 in 2001; treated in New York City, NY.)

Hints for Dealing with Hair Loss

- Buy some pretty or funky headscarves and hats. Experiment with different styles that you like.
- Try a wig. Wigs are versatile and can range from the subtle to the outrageous. If you want your wig to look like your old hair, it's a good idea to purchase it before your hair loss is extensive. That way you can match the color and style more easily. You may even be able to get a tax credit for the wig as a medical expense, or it may be covered by your health insurance.
- Use this opportunity to experiment with different looks that you might not otherwise try (have you ever wondered what you'd look like with a bright purple Mohawk? Why not find out?).
- Ask you doctor about a controversial therapy called scalp hypothermia, a process by which the scalp is chilled before and during treatments. Be aware, however, that there is disagreement among professionals as to whether this really helps.

Adapted from the Canadian Cancer Society's booklet "Chemotherapy and You" and the American Cancer Society's webpage "Understanding Chemotherapy."

TEMPORARY MENOPAUSE

Chemotherapy often affects your menstrual cycle. Some women experience irregular periods while other women stop having periods altogether (if you had a hysterectomy, you won't have periods at all anymore, since the uterus has been removed). Some women also experience other symptoms commonly associated with menopause, such as hot flashes, mood swings and changes in body shape. These changes are often temporary and thus are part of what's been dubbed "temporary menopause" or "chemically induced menopause." These changes tend to disappear after treatment. When they persist, however, they signal the onset of premature menopause. You may want to discuss estrogen replacement therapy with your doctor if you find you've entered premature menopause.

Some of the women we spoke with experienced temporary menopause:

> "Didn't have any periods while I was on chemo—it was great!" (Diagnosed at 30 in 1997; treated in Sheffield, UK.)

> "I continued to menstruate [while] having EMA, but when on EMA-CO, after the second treatment I no longer did. I remember having night sweats and terrible hot flashes for several months. I ended up having the hysterectomy so that was that! Now it's permanent menopause!" (Diagnosed at 41 in 1999; treated in Memphis, TN, then Fort Lauderdale, FL.)

Vaginal Dryness

The lining of your vagina is constantly shed and replaced. For this reason chemotherapy drugs can have an effect on vaginal tissues. Some women experience vaginal itching, burning or dryness. This in turn can cause a diminished interest in sex (see chapter 7 for more information on sex and intimacy).

There are several ways to deal with vaginal dryness. Some women don't find it to be a problem, except when they want to engage in intercourse. For these women a water-based lubricant such as KY Jelly or Eros can be helpful (these are sold at pharmacies and sex shops). Other women are bothered by dryness and in this case a long-lasting product such as Replens is more helpful. Replens keeps the vagina moist for about eight hours. Finally, you may want to ask your doctor about prescribing a cream that contains estrogen. This will also help you maintain a moist vagina for a long period of time. I am still bothered by this at least once a month. It gets so itchy down there, and the more you scratch, the more it itches. It hurts too. I can't even walk or sit still without having to "do something" about it. I've used Replens and a prescription estrogen cream that works after a few days. I've also tried lubricant, and that works somewhat. For instant temporary relief I've used Vaseline or even just a plain lotion (like Vaseline Intensive Care). If I have any hair growing down there, I have to shave it off because the "pricklies" are just too irritating.

Hot Flashes

Physical signs of hot flashes range from a feeling of warmth in the face and upper body, to simultaneous sweating and chills, anxiety, tension, tingling in the fingers, dizziness and nausea. Researchers believe hot flashes are caused by a decrease in estrogen, which causes the hypothalamus (which controls both body temperature and sex hormones) to malfunction. Vegetarians are less likely to have hot flashes. Women who are 10 percent or more over their "ideal weight" are less likely to have severe hot flashes. This is because fatty tissue acts as a "factory" to convert androstenedione, an adrenal hormone, into estrone. Women who exercise vigorously have fewer severe flashes as compared to non-exercisers. Relaxation training, involving slow, deep abdominal breathing, has also been demonstrated to reduce the frequency of hot flashes. Stress may increase the frequency or intensity of flashes, and so will a high room temperature or warm climate. Women subject to hot flashes are better off in cool temperatures with lots of circulating air.

Hot flashes are so annoying. Having to put on a sweater, then take it off, then put it on again. It sucked when I was talking to people and had to interrupt them not once, but five or more times. Even trying to pay attention while going through the hot flash was a challenge, trying to cool down and sweating like crazy. I used to wake up in the middle of the night and change my pajamas because the ones I was wearing were soaked. Yep, it sucked.

Some of the women we spoke with experienced hot flashes, but said there wasn't much they could do about them:

> "Yes, I felt as if someone were spraying me with fire, up and down my body, while I broke out into a sweat, feeling dizzy and faint. Wearing the wig didn't help, in 95 degree Florida. It was difficult to sleep; nothing helped really." (Diagnosed at 41 in 1999; treated in Memphis, TN, then Fort Lauderdale, FL.)

> "I only experienced hot flashes after my ovaries were removed and I began menopause. I would start to feel real hot, then my face would become red and I would start to sweat. During the night, I often had to change bedclothes two or three times. Winter was the worst because I started out in a flannel nightgown and ended up nude!" (Diagnosed at 27 in 1973; treated in Southampton, NY, and New York City, NY.)

Tips to Control Hot Flashes

- Avoid synthetic clothing and bedding because it traps perspiration.
- Avoid clothing with high necks and long sleeves.
- Dress in layers.
- Keep cold drinks handy.
- Cut down on, or quit smoking.
- Avoid caffeine, alcohol, spicy foods, sugars and large meals.
- Eat soy-based products and other foods that contain phytoestrogens such as yams.
- Discuss taking vitamin E supplements with your doctor.
- Exercise to improve your circulation.
- Reduce exposure to the sun.
- Ask your physician about Effexor, an antidepressant drug that in low doses (usually 37.5 mg, twice a day) may help some women with hot flashes. This might be an option if you are really bothered.

Adapted from the Canadian Cancer Society's booklet "Chemotherapy and You" and the American Cancer Society's webpage "Understanding Chemotherapy."

OTHER SIDE EFFECTS

There are various other side effects associated with chemotherapy. These are usually temporary. Like the side effects mentioned above, some of them are caused when the chemotherapy drugs prevent normal cells from dividing and replacing themselves as needed. Others, such as fluid retention, are caused by the large amounts of fluid that are introduced into your body via the IV. Still others (such as sleep disorders) are caused by the added stress of undergoing chemotherapy and the manner in which this affects your life.

Muscles and Nerves

Some chemotherapy drugs may have an effect on your muscles or nerves. You may notice that your muscles seem weaker or that they're achy and sore. Some patients experience a ringing sensation in their ears (called tinnitus). This ringing sensation is caused by damage to the nerve endings. Some patients report that their balance is affected by chemotherapy. Other patients experience a tingling or burning sensation in their hands or feet, similar to when these limbs "fall asleep." You may find that some tasks, such as doing up buttons or opening jars, are more difficult because of the tingling.

To protect yourself from injury you should be aware of these sensations. Move slowly if your balance is off and use handrails when climbing stairs. If your fingers feel numb, be extra cautious when using sharp tools or near hot items.

These side effects are usually temporary, but you should report them to your doctor at your next visit.

I've experienced all of these symptoms (and still am experiencing some of them)! I used to get muscle aches to the extent that I felt like I'd been in a major car accident and that I was bruised all over. I wasn't, but that's how I felt. If I moved it was very painful and if anyone touched me it was even more painful. I still have a constant ringing in my ears, which I've learned to deal with and ignore (for the most part). It's like the ringing that you get after you get home from a bar or a concert and you're back in a quiet place. Except it doesn't go away. One of the chemo drugs that I was given (cisplatin) caused hearing loss as well. I can't hear certain high-pitched sounds (like the beep when the thermometer is done; I have to wait until the Celsius sign stops flashing). My balance has been affected slightly, although not so much that I have to be constantly careful. I have tingling in my feet (which causes me a lot of pain as well) and my fingertips are worse. Now all I feel is numbness in my fingertips (kind of like when your skin is so dry you can't really "feel" what you're touching). This is constant and irreversible.

Urinary Tract

Some chemotherapy drugs may change the color of your urine. For example, methotrexate may turn your urine a bright yellow color. You may also notice a different odor to your urine. Don't be alarmed.

Drink plenty of fluids to prevent urinary tract infection and to keep your urine flowing. Go to the bathroom frequently to prevent a build-up of urine in your bladder. Since chemotherapy makes you prone to infection, it's important to go pee frequently to avoid a bladder or kidney infection. Wipe from front to back after using the bathroom to avoid spreading germs from your anus to your urethra. And since some chemotherapy drugs affect your kidney and bladder function, you'll need to ask your doctor about signs to watch out for.

I used to get bladder infections frequently when I was younger, but ended up getting one while on treatment, and had to stay in the hospital for a week to try to get rid of it. Bladder infections can be very uncomfortable and/or painful while just sitting or walking around. To ease the pain, drink some cranberry juice. You can also use an over-the-counter urinary pain medicine such as Pyridium, Azo Standard or the generic name phenazopyridine, which eases the pain (but will turn your urine a bright red/orange color).

One of the women we interviewed reported urinary tract infections:

> "Bladder infection? Often during [the] chemo years. What helped me feel better? Drinking lots of water [and other] fluids." (Diagnosed at 36 in 1993; treated in Manila, Philippines, and Kuala Lumpur, Malaysia.)

Fluid Retention (Edema and Lymphedema)

Lymphedema is the accumulation of lymph in the fatty tissues of the body. Lymph is the fluid that circulates in your body to keep your tissues moist. In lymphedema, your body's lymphatic system fails to return the lymphatic fluid to the blood. Patients who are obese or have poor nutrition are particularly at risk for developing lymphedema. Lymphedema is markedly increased in women after removal of the lymph nodes during surgery or following radiation to the lymph nodes. Women may also experience edema, wherein extra fluid accumulates in the tissues because it leaks out of the blood vessels. This is more frequent with women with malnutrition and poor blood protein levels. The symptoms of edema and lymphedema are a feeling of tightness in your hands and feet (you may notice that your rings get too tight, or that shoes and gloves no longer fit), as well as decreased strength, pain, aching or heaviness, and redness or swelling in the hands and feet. Some of the swelling and bloating may be caused by the large amount of fluid that is being pumped into your body with each chemotherapy treatment. Your fluid intake is also likely to be quite a bit higher since you'll be drinking more water than average.

Sometimes the hormonal changes that are associated with temporary menopause may make you feel bloated. Menopausal women have reported feelings of swollen hands, feet, face and abdomen. If swelling is a problem, cut down on the amount of salt in your diet. If the problem develops suddenly (you blow up like a balloon) or if the problem is severe, call your doctor immediately.

Some of the women we spoke with experienced bloating:

> "Yes, very bad. And it was very uncomfortable. I couldn't fit in any of my clothes." (Diagnosed at 24 in 2001; treated in New York City, NY.)

> "I drank as much liquid as possible to keep me flushed out, so I did feel bloated at times." (Diagnosed at 41 in 1999; treated in Memphis, TN, then Fort Lauderdale, FL.)

Helpful Hints for Dealing with Edema and Lymphedema
- Exercise. Mobility helps the functioning of the lymphatic system.
- Keep your hands and/or feet elevated above the heart whenever possible.
- Avoid rapid circular movements.
- Avoid applying tight bandages. Use gauze instead of tape bandages.
- Avoid getting a needle or IV in the affected extremity.
- Avoid using heating pads or ice packs on the affected limb.
- Avoid prolonged work using the affected limb.
- Wear loose clothing (avoid elastics) and jewelry.
- Carry your handbag with the unaffected arm (or get someone else to carry it if both arms are affected). Avoid wearing heavy backpacks that may put stress on the shoulder.
- Don't use blood pressure cuffs on the affected arm.
- Avoid wearing pantyhose or tights.
- Don't sit in one position for a prolonged period of time. Try to change positions at least every 30 minutes.
- Be aware that your sensation in the affected limb may be diminished. Be careful around hot or sharp items.
- Massage the arm or leg, starting at the hand or foot and working towards the torso.
- Use compression garments if recommended by your doctor. Be aware however that these should only be used under medical supervision.

Adapted from the Canadian Cancer Society's booklet "Chemotherapy and You" and the American Cancer Society's webpage "Understanding Chemotherapy."

Sleep Disorders

While about 12 to 25 percent of the general population has sleep disorders, it has been estimated that 45 percent of people with cancer experience sleep disturbances. Poor sleep can negatively impact your mood and make the emotional side effects of treatment (see pages 152–159) worse. Sleep disorders can also be an early signal of developing delirium. Choriocarcinoma patients and women receiving chemotherapy to treat their GTN often experience insomnia (the inability to begin sleep) as well as a tendency to wake up easily once they have fallen asleep. Furthermore, many of the side effects of chemotherapy (pain, hot flashes, digestive problems and difficulty breathing) have been found to contribute to sleep disorders even among people who don't have a disease. If you were in the hospital your sleep was probably interrupted several times a night when the nurse came in to check on you. If you grew accustomed to this cycle of interruptions, you may have difficulty getting back to a normal sleeping pattern when you return home.

Lack of exercise further contributes to sleep problems. Add to that the anxiety (another cause of sleeping difficulty) of having a life-threatening illness, and it's a wonder that chemotherapy patients get any sleep at all!

I had difficulty sleeping, especially when I was first diagnosed and after the first few treatments. Getting adjusted to such a major change in your life as well as reacting and dealing with the chemo drugs in your body takes a toll on you mentally. I was prescribed a very mild sleeping pill that seemed not to kick in until morning, so I'd sleep the day away (which I often did later on anyway). So, I quit taking those. What did help eventually was self-hypnosis (I had cassette tapes from a hypnotist that I played) or wearing the earplugs Meredith had given me.

Helpful Hints for Getting Some Sleep

- Get a relaxing massage of your back, head, scalp, shoulders, hands and feet.
- Keep your bedding wrinkle- and crumb-free.
- Stay warm in bed, with enough blankets.
- Avoid drinking before bed, so that you won't wake up to pee. Try to use the bathroom before bed.
- Wear earplugs to block out noise.
- Eat foods high in tryptophan (e.g., turkey and milk).

- Avoid caffeine and chocolate, especially before bed.
- Exercise no less than two hours before bed but also try to exercise daily.
- Try to keep a regular bedtime schedule.
- Ask your doctor to minimize and coordinate bedside contacts while you're an inpatient. Telling staff about your sleep difficulties will make them more understanding.

Adapted from the Canadian Cancer Society's booklet "Chemotherapy and You" and the American Cancer Society's webpage "Understanding Chemotherapy."

Delirium

Delirium is characterized by disturbances in cognitive function. Delirium is defined as a condition of extreme mental (and usually motor) excitement marked by defective perception, impaired memory and a rapid succession of confused and unconnected ideas, often with illusions and hallucinations. Delirium needs immediate medical attention. The disturbances in cognitive function can include: disturbances of attention, thinking, perception, judgment, emotion and memory, as well as problems organizing activities and difficulty with multi-tasking. It can also be accompanied by disorientation. Tasks seem more difficult to complete and require increased effort, and you lose the ability to do things on "auto-pilot." Delirium can cause fatigue, since everything you do takes more effort. Fatigue, in turn, can also increase delirium.

Delirium can be a direct result of cancer if there are tumors present in the brain. The chemotherapeutic drugs used to treat GTN can also cause delirium. Methotrexate, cisplatin and vincristine have all been linked to delirium. Furthermore, opioids used to control pain may increase levels of delirium. Although some of the symptoms of delirium may be permanent, delirium is largely reversible and often disappears after treatment.

Helpful Hints to Deal with Delirium

- Surround yourself with familiar objects. Keep a clock and calendar visible.
- Educate your family about delirium. Many family members find this side effect frightening.

- Avoid driving and operating heavy machinery.
- Write things down to help you remember. Don't rely too heavily on this method, however, because memory improves with practice. As you get better try to write things down less often until you memory has improved.

Adapted from the Canadian Cancer Society's booklet "Chemotherapy and You" and the American Cancer Society's webpage "Understanding Chemotherapy."

Chemo-Brain

Sometimes going through chemotherapy treatment can cause a milder form of impaired thinking. This form is much less severe than delirium, but may still cause patients to forget things and feel "out of sorts." Patients refer to this side effect as "chemo brain." After a few treatments, I noticed that there were days I couldn't concentrate long enough to read a sentence, let alone a paragraph out of the medical journals we'd collected. I'd lose my thoughts in the middle of a sentence, or even before I spoke! I used to be able to remember where everyone had last put things (like TJ and his dang hat!) and now I couldn't even remember where I'd put my purse. It really bothered me, and still does, even though it's better, because I was so dependent on my memory. Now I can't even remember what happened a week ago!

Here is what the some of the women we spoke to reported about chemo brain:

> "Yes I experienced it, and I still do. It's very upsetting to me because I feel stupid. But I'm learning to write a lot of things down now, to help me, and [I've adopted] little techniques here and there to assist with it. My doc told me that exercising the brain helps this, so that's what I'm doing now. I'm also going to be starting occupational therapy in the next month to help with this." (Diagnosed at 24 in 2001; treated in New York City, NY.)

> "I suffered for years with "chemo brain" as they now call it. I had both short and long term memory loss. I lost all memory of everything up to two minutes ago. I asked questions over and over again. I was told: "You just asked me that two minutes ago!" Well, I was sorry but I couldn't remember even asking the question, let alone [getting an] answer. I remembered my family, my husband, my sons, and my closest friends, but I forgot everything else.

Gradually, however, my memory returned. I'd say it took about four years." (Diagnosed at 27 in 1973; treated in Southampton, NY, and New York City, NY.)

Hypercalcemia (excess calcium in the blood)

Hypercalcemia occurs in 10 to 20 percent of chemotherapy patients, but is very rare in GTN patients. In cancer, hypercalcemia can be caused by bone metastases or a reaction to certain drugs (some diurectics). In healthy individuals the kidneys filter calcium from the blood. In chemotherapy patients, kidney function may be compromised by the powerful drugs. Furthermore, dehydration, immobility, vomiting and diarrhea contribute to hypercalcemia. Drinking plenty of water and juice can help prevent hypercalcemia. Cisplatin (one of the drugs used in choriocarcinoma chemotherapy) protects against hypercalcemia.

Hypercalcemia can be life-threatening, so it's an important side effect to watch out for. However, it's difficult to detect because the symptoms are general and may be attributed to other problems. The symptoms of hypercalcemia are: malaise and fatigue (the most commonly reported), anorexia, pain, constipation, nausea and vomiting, delirium or stupor, headache, dehydration and thirst, and diminished sweating. Your doctor will test for hypercalcemia by looking at your blood sample analysis.

Flu-Like Symptoms

Chemotherapy patients often report that they feel like they have the flu after treatment. The symptoms may last a few hours or a few days.

Some of the women we spoke with reported feeling flu-like symptoms:

"Yes. What helped me feel better? Analgesics and antipyretics." (Diagnosed at 36 in 1993; treated in Manila, Philippines, and Kuala Lumpur, Malaysia.)

"I believe the -CO part gave me flu-like symptoms, but [it wasn't] too bad. I felt achy from too much Neupogen®, and would take a Tylenol to alleviate the bone pain." (Diagnosed at 41 in 1999; treated in Memphis, TN, then Fort Lauderdale, FL.)

THE EMOTIONAL SIDE EFFECTS OF CHEMOTHERAPY TREATMENTS

Many chemotherapy patients (25 to 40 percent) experience emotional effects from treatments as well as physical effects. This is not surprising. Being told you have a serious disease is very frightening. You may find that you're reevaluating your life's path and your relationships. You may also feel confused and uncertain about what's happening to you.

When I was first diagnosed, I had no clue what was ahead of me. I really didn't know how much life would change, and how my cancer would affect me, not to mention everybody around me. I was so mad at the doctor who diagnosed me because I knew it should have been caught earlier. I was mad at myself for not pushing for a better answer from the doctor. And I was scared. *I have cancer*, I kept thinking. I didn't know anyone who had cancer and I had no clue what it meant. Or, for that matter, how I actually got it. But I knew I had to deal with it. I kept thinking and hoping and wishing that it wouldn't be long until I'd recovered and was back to my old life. And when this didn't happen, thoughts and emotions started running through my head like crazy. I wanted to talk about everything I was thinking and feeling, but TJ wasn't ready to talk about anything bad—especially death and what was going to happen to him and the kids if I died. So, I didn't talk about it much—at first.

Feelings of fear, anxiety and anger are normal and are experienced by many patients. It's important to remember that you're not alone. Try to accept that chemotherapy treatments will temporarily affect your lifestyle. You'll have to power down somewhat, and take it easy until you recover. Some people who lead busy lives find this makes them restless. Others feel like they're missing out on their youth.

Remember that by readjusting your attitude (as well as your activities) you may be able to handle these emotions better than you think. Many people find that talking out their feelings is useful. In fact emotional challenges associated with chemotherapy are so common there is a new branch of psychology (called psycho-oncology) dedicated exclusively to studying the feelings common to cancer patients. You may want to talk to a therapist who specializes in cancer psychotherapy. Or you may know a clergy member you trust. You may also want to join a support group to talk with other patients. (See the resource list for places to turn for support.) You may have a close friend or family member with whom you can talk openly about your emotions and fears. Whatever works for you is the right approach to take. Remember that everyone needs extra support when they're going through a life-changing event like GTN therapy.

It's very tough to stay positive throughout treatment. There will be days where you think you can't handle being sick anymore, mentally or physically. I'd have a huge cry whenever I felt this way, and though it didn't take the pain away it felt good to get it out. Sometimes I found it really hard to relax, and at these times, crying didn't help at all. I wanted to be my old self again, with no pain and no sickness. And I knew this wasn't going to happen, which made me more miserable. I didn't want to talk to anyone. I just stayed in bed most of the time. If I got up, I'd take my frustrations out on everyone—including those helping out. I'm sure I was a huge joy to live with! At the time I remember thinking that it would never end, that I couldn't even see the light at the end of the tunnel. Everything—how long treatments lasted, what my counts were like—was a waiting game. This made everything that much harder, because I didn't have an inkling of when any of it would end.

I found that having help around the house really helped me stay positive, because I didn't have to deal with the stress of caring for my family as well as keeping the house clean. Another positive influence came from family and friends. Everyone I knew kept telling me that I'd beat the disease, that I was young and that I'd been through a lot in my life already. They told me that I was a very strong woman. This made me *believe* I could beat it. I had to: I had a family who needed me, and friends and relatives who I cared about a great deal. I had to prove to them that I was strong.

You may actually find that you become a source of strength, support and inspiration to your friends. Meredith reports that she was amazed by my positive attitude, and that she often felt more supported by me!

One of the women we spoke with stressed the importance of finding a support group to help you with emotional reactions to diagnosis and treatment.

> "Support groups are so important, and [they provide] a way to share what you're going through. This book will be wonderful as a reference or guide, just knowing someone else has been there and gone through it!" (Diagnosed at 41 in 1999; treated in Memphis, TN, then Fort Lauderdale, FL.)

Tips to Make Life Easier During Chemotherapy

- Make a list of techniques you used to deal with stressful situations in the past. These may be able to help you now.
- Eat well to maintain your strength. Being undernourished affects your mood.
- Exercise and get out of the house. This will also help to increase your appetite.
- Keep a journal or diary. Sometimes writing things down helps you to get a bit of distance and gain perspective on how you're feeling.
- Do the things that are important to you first. Don't let chemotherapy rob you of your social life. Leave less important things for later—only if you feel up to it.
- Set realistic goals and don't be too hard on yourself. Do the activities that you can do, but know when to delegate activities to others.
- Plan activities for the days when you feel best.

Adapted from the National Cancer Institute's webpage "Eating Hints For Cancer Patients," the Canadian Cancer Society's booklet "Chemotherapy and You," the Canadian Cancer Society's booklet "Taking Time" and the American Cancer Society's webpage "Understanding Chemotherapy."

ANXIETY

Anxiety is a normal response to receiving a GTN diagnosis. Many patients report feelings of anxiety while they're waiting for the results of diagnostic tests. Anxiety can heighten your experience of other side effects such as pain or sleeplessness. Anxiety can also interfere with your ability to absorb information, making communication with your doctor more difficult.

Studies have found that hormone-producing diseases (of which choriocarcinoma and other forms of GTN are examples) are linked to an increase in feelings of anxiety when compared to other types of disease. I was very anxious—especially in the beginning, when everything was new to me. The waiting game, the realization of the diagnosis, and starting chemo drugs for the first time was very overwhelming. Not to mention frustrating, which just adds to the anxiety. You have so much to remember in so little time. It's a whole new life. You're going through test after test and speaking to nurses, doctors and more nurses. Every one of them has something to tell you, advice to give, things for you to do, etc. Plus, you're being pumped full of drugs—the names of which you can't spell let alone pronounce—and you have to take what home, when? Ugh!

Here is what we heard from chorio survivors about anxiety:

> "Yes, lots. [So] much it interfered with daily activities, [and I] had one week where I did nothing but cry. Prozac and counseling helped. [As did my] hCG coming down every week!" (Diagnosed at 30 in 1997; treated in Sheffield, UK.)

> "[I was anxious] all the time! I analyzed everything: my lab reports, my latest hCG reading, how the nurse looked at me, etc. I tried to talk about it with my husband, mom and sister, who helped tremendously. The chemo nurse helped me a lot by simply answering my questions "straight," but with kindness. I never took any pills for it or anything, just muddled through." (Diagnosed at 41 in 1999; treated in Memphis, TN, then Fort Lauderdale, FL.)

> "I just felt nervous that my life was never going to return to normal. I tried not to let it interfere with my daily activities. But sometimes when I was alone I remember crying about it and asking God: *Why me?* He always seemed to answer: *Because I knew you could handle it.*" (Diagnosed at 27 in 1973; treated in Southampton, NY, and New York City, NY.)

Tips for Coping with Anxiety
- Confront your fears directly. Ask your doctor about things that are making you anxious. Talk about your fears with a loved one or friend.
- Join a support group to discuss your fears.
- Try to view the situation as a problem to be solved, or as a challenge to be overcome. Then think of all the challenges you've met in the past!
- Get complete information.
- Try to be flexible and take things as they come.
- Think of major events or tasks as a series of smaller tasks. Take pride in accomplishing each step.

Adapted from the Canadian Cancer Society's booklet "Chemotherapy and You," the Canadian Cancer Society's booklet "Taking Time" and the American Cancer Society's webpage "Understanding Chemotherapy."

STRESS

Stress is a normal part of life. Everyone has experienced stress from time to time. Stress can even be good for you (it can motivate you to make changes!). However, too much stress can compromise your health. Feeling chronically stressed can interfere with your immune system, something that chemotherapy patients need to avoid. This is because stress causes a "flight or fight" response in your body. Under normal circumstances this response is used to deal with an emergency situation. Energy resources in your body are diverted away from your immune system in order to deal with the imminent danger. In chronic stress, this immune suppression can be dangerous. Studies have shown that patients with high levels of stress take longer to recover from chemotherapy treatments.

Recent studies have even suggested that the experience of cancer is so stressful that cancer patients may be at risk for post-traumatic stress disorder. However, everyone responds to stress differently.

I was really stressed, especially when they had to change my chemo protocol a couple of times because the previous one wasn't working anymore, and my counts weren't dropping at all. I get really stressed when my counts go up. Here are two other women's experiences of stress:

> "Sure [I was stressed]... most of the stress came from not very much information out there to help, and the incompetence of some of the nurses and doctors, who were doing the best they could, I imagine, but [who] were overworked, etc. Also, projecting what the future held was stressful, and of course dealing with insurance claims and money problems added to the pot!" (Diagnosed at 41 in 1999; treated in Memphis, TN, then Fort Lauderdale, FL.)

> "I think stress wasn't a word used back then, but *pressure* was. I felt pressure to do everything as if nothing had happened to me. I was to cook, clean, wash, iron, take care of the kids, etc., as if I hadn't just been sick and gone through hell. I'm surprised I didn't have a nervous breakdown. I think I have always kept it bottled up inside of me. I never found a release for it." (Diagnosed at 27 in 1973; treated in Southampton, NY, and New York City, NY.)

Tips for Coping with Stress

- Some people report that herbal supplements help with stress. However it's important to check with your doctor before taking these drugs since they may interact with chemotherapy.
- Add some aromatherapy oils to your bath, or heat some in a clay pot. Oils that reduce stress include: ylang ylang, neroli, jasmine, orange blossom, cedarwood, lavender (a few drops on your pillow will also help you sleep), chamomile, marjoram, geranium, patchouli, rose, sage, clary sage, and sandalwood.
- Practice yoga or meditation.
- Get some time to yourself.
- Pamper yourself. I thought it was quite funny when one day as everyone was leaving my stepson Tragean informed me that he'd decided to stay home and "take care" of me. I mentioned to him that he could pamper me. Since we had a one-year-old at home, he was instantly thinking differently than I was, and said: "I'm not going to put a diaper on you mom!"
- Have someone give you a massage.
- Surround yourself with supportive people and avoid interpersonal stress. When you're surrounded by people who take energy from you rather than give you energy in the form of support, the result is more stress in you life. By doing a serious reevaluation of your personal relationships, you may be able to find more energy and reduce the amount of stress in your life.
- Forgive. An unresolved conflict with someone can increase your levels of stress. The emotional weight you carry when you think about the conflict increases blood pressure, stress hormones, heart rate, perspiration, and muscle tension. This can increase your experience of treatment side effects. Forgiveness doesn't mean excusing bad behavior, but it does mean that you're prepared to move forward and let go of bitterness. Forgiveness is healthier for you, and chances are the person with whom you're engaged in conflict would either welcome your forgiveness or, if they're also nursing a grudge, would, deep down, want to forgive you too.
- Don't be too hard on yourself. Don't forget that it is also important to forgive yourself.

- Cry a little. Human tears contain high levels of stress hormone, which is one reason why people who cry tend to have less stress than those who don't cry.
- Laugh! Laugh a lot! Laughter is a great stress reliever. Watch a funny movie, or invite a friend over who makes you laugh.

Adapted from Dr. M. Sara Rosenthal's The Breast Sourcebook *(Lowell House: 1997), the National Cancer Institute's webpage "Eating Hints For Cancer Patients," the Canadian Cancer Society's booklet "Chemotherapy and You," the Canadian Cancer Society's booklet "Taking Time" and the American Cancer Society's webpage "Understanding Chemotherapy."*

DEPRESSION

Depression is thought to affect between 15 and 23 percent of chemotherapy patients. Families of people undergoing chemotherapy are also at risk for depression. Depression is an understandable reaction, since GTN and its treatment can often disrupt your life plans, cause changes in your self-image and self-esteem, as well as changes in your social roles and lifestyle. Furthermore, if you have to take time off work you may have financial constraints that add to depression. Depression is understandable, but prolonged depression is not normal and should be treated.

Some patients blame themselves and think things like "I brought this on myself" or "God is punishing me" or "I'm letting my family down." These kinds of thoughts are not a problem if they occur only occasionally. But if these thoughts persist despite evidence to the contrary, they may signal that you're depressed.

Depression can affect the functioning of your immune system. When you feel low, your whole body slows down. Studies have found that patients who had prolonged episodes of depression while undergoing chemotherapy had reduced survival rates when compared with patients who were able to keep a positive attitude.

If you feel depressed, you may benefit from psychotherapy. If your doctor prescribes antidepressant medication, take the drugs exactly as directed. And if you want to stop taking this medication, it's best to consult with your doctor, since some drugs need to be discontinued gradually. Moreover, suddenly stopping some antidepressant medications can be fatal.

I believe I was depressed for quite some time when I was sick. But I wasn't given anything (medically) to help me through it, so I just hoped for the best and for the treatment to work. I'm sure that if I hadn't started feeling better when I did I would have been given medication to help me through it.

Some of the women we interviewed reported feeling depressed:

> "I think I remained positive through most of the illness until after the hysterectomy. I almost asked my doctor for anti-depressants. My aunt had a friend going through chemo for breast cancer and she was on Zoloft and said it was helpful. I never did [ask], and got out of it in a month or so." (Diagnosed at 41 in 1999; treated in Memphis, TN, then Fort Lauderdale, FL.)

> "I guess you could have called my crying spells depression. I'd wait until no one was around to hear me and then I'd sit alone somewhere and just cry until I couldn't cry anymore. Maybe the release helped me feel better, [or helped me] to go on. That and my boys. Anytime I looked at them it helped me feel like I had a purpose." (Diagnosed at 27 in 1973; treated in Southampton, NY, and New York City, NY.)

NUTRITION AND CHEMOTHERAPY

Eating well is always vital to maintaining good health. And it's particularly important during chemotherapy, because you need to maintain stamina throughout your treatment. Patients who eat a variety of foods that contain vitamins, minerals and proteins are better able to deal with the side effects of chemotherapy.

Some studies have found that as many as 40 percent to 80 percent of chemotherapy patients have some degree of clinical malnutrition. Malnutrition reduces your immune system's ability to work properly. As we noted earlier in this chapter, it's particularly important for a chemotherapy patient to protect her immune system, as it can be damaged by low blood cell counts. Malnourished patients take longer to recover from surgery. They're less able to tolerate chemotherapy and may require longer breaks between cycles. Furthermore, malnourished patients experience more severe side effects from treatments. Malnutrition contributes to fatigue and diminishes quality of life. It results in longer periods of hospitalization and lowered survival rates.

Some patients become malnourished as a result of the physical side effects from chemotherapy (e.g., feeling full, taste changes, constipation, diarrhea, nausea, etc.) Other patients become malnourished because they're unable to purchase food (they may not have enough money, since they may have had to leave work, or they may just feel too "worn out" to do the shopping). Different cultures perceive the relationship between food and illness in different ways, and sometimes a patient's cultural background contributes to malnutrition. Finally, many chemotherapy patients report that they're simply too tired to eat. Fatigue can decrease your desire to prepare meals even if you are hungry. Add digestive problems and loss of appetite to the mix and it is a wonder that chemotherapy patients eat at all!

Foods rich in protein are especially important to eat during treatment since your body needs protein to repair tissues that have been damaged by chemotherapy. However, if you don't take in enough calories, your body will be forced to use protein for energy that could otherwise have been used for repairs. Furthermore, many "forbidden foods" (such as ice cream) actually help with side effects. Since chemotherapy tends to make you lose weight you can look at this as an opportunity to enjoy the foods you might otherwise avoid!

When I first started treatments, I didn't have a problem with eating at all. Actually, I ate more. Then, the more treatments I did, the harder it was to eat. The smell of food made me sick to my stomach. There were also days where all I wanted to do was sleep so I wouldn't have to feel so sick. And eating would just make me feel worse. On days when I felt really hungry my husband TJ made me Kraft Dinner. I'd eat two or three bites out of it and not be able to eat any more. And I'd have to force even those bites down. The supplements, for me, had a real tinny taste so I couldn't force them down at all. I was malnourished. I hated the taste of most foods. It wasn't enjoyable to eat *or* drink. Any time I drank water, I'd have to run to the bathroom, because I couldn't keep it down. Or, I'd feel even worse for a couple of hours. In short, I've experienced all of the reactions mentioned in this chapter. Some were a lot harder to deal with than others, but for the most part, they all got frustrating.

We've offered a lot of pointers herein. I know it's hard to keep up with everything you're being told—especially when you're feeling like crap. Find what works best for you in the beginning; you may have to change it as your treatment progresses. Try your best at eating and get help if you find you aren't able to eat or drink anything.

CHAPTER 7

PERSONAL RELATIONSHIPS AND INTIMACY

HOW TO DEAL WITH YOUR FRIENDS AND FAMILY

Families play an important role in caregiving for GTN patients. This has become increasingly true in recent years, as chemotherapy treatments have improved, reducing the need for long stays in the hospital. And it means that most of your recovery will be done at home—so your family will be enlisted to help and to facilitate. Family members provide as much as 80 percent of the care for patients undergoing chemotherapy. Women often play a central role in the daily management of family life. When you find out you have GTN your ability to perform this role may be limited; therefore the GTN diagnosis will have an impact on your whole family.

This section of the book looks at personal relationships and how to make these a source of strength, rather than allowing them to become an energy drain. Going through the experience of GTN will demand a lot of understanding and sympathy from everyone involved. You'll have to deal with your own fears as well as the fears of your family. And you'll have to remember that sometimes people behave badly when they're under stress. If a family member has an angry outburst, he or she may be expressing frustration at the situation, rather than anger at you. We sometimes vent our frustrations on the ones we love. Although this can be painful, it can also show us how much we're trusted.

This chapter contains information on how you can cope with friends and family. It also includes information aimed at friends and family, since they'll need to cope with choriocarcinoma or GTN as well.

HUSBANDS AND PARTNERS

Being married sure has its ups and downs. My husband, TJ, sure gets on my nerves some days (as I do his!). But all in all, it comes down to love, trust, communication, and living each day as it is. You are in it together: throughout the diagnosis, treatment and anything else that may happen before, during and afterwards. I was so scared when I was called in to the doctor's office and told to bring my husband. TJ, trying not to think of the bad, just kept reassuring me. He tried to be so strong throughout the whole ordeal, and to be there for me as much as possible—or as much as he was allowed to be.

TJ told us his view: "We've been married for almost three years now, and we sure have gone through a lot. When Tara and I were told that she had a rare type of cancer, the seriousness of it didn't really register. We were told it was a *type* of cancer, so it took me a while to clue in that it really was *cancer*, and was actually something serious. It wasn't until she had all the complications with the first chemo that I realized what was going on."

We asked a couple of our women with chorio how their husbands found out about their diagnosis. Here is what they said:

> "I got a call from my family practitioner telling me the results of the biopsy. I called my husband right away at work. I just came out and told him "I have cancer," then told him about [the details], the little that I did know at the time. I was thinking: "I can't leave my kids!" I was also thinking about all the things I/we weren't going to be able to do: nursing my baby, family vacation, new car, landscaping, etc." (Diagnosed in 2001; treated in Minnesota.)

> "My husband and I were called in to meet with my doctors in the doctors' lounge of our local hospital. It was there that they explained to us that I was "very sick." That in the month since my operation a spot had shown up on my chest X-ray. That they had conferred with some doctors in the city (New York) and that I was to be admitted by 2 p.m. that day. We packed a bag and drove over 100 miles to the hospital. No one really gave us a chance to think about it. It wasn't until later that day that we even had a chance to discuss what had happened. I was very nervous and scared." (Diagnosed at 27 in 1973; treated in Southampton, NY, and New York City, NY.)

Sex

Many GTN patients report changes in sexual desire during (and sometimes after) therapy. These changes in desire are often caused by physical and emotional changes as well as changes in self-image.

If you've had a hysterectomy, you may feel less feminine. Many women think of their uterus, their periods and their fertility as fundamental to their sexuality. Some women report difficulty becoming aroused after a hysterectomy. However, other women see the hysterectomy as a relief from the pain and heavy bleeding of menstruation, the end of which opens up a new and freer sexual life. Intercourse is usually permitted after six weeks; however, some women prefer to wait longer. After a period of abstinence, reestablishing sexual contact may be difficult (see pages 165–166 for more information on reestablishing contact).

Some women report that their vagina feels tight or that they experience pain during intercourse because of tender scar tissues. Sometimes hysterectomy, chemotherapy and/or radiation therapy can shrink the vagina. Sex is actually recommended as a method of maintaining the vagina's shape. Your vagina may be dry due to the side effects of chemotherapy (see page 142), making intercourse painful. Sometimes you may want sex, but your body doesn't seem to be willing.

I found that before being diagnosed, with my intermittent bleeding for nine months, it was really hard to get "in the mood," because I'd started to feel really gross, and had also started to get angry that the bleeding hadn't completely stopped. Not all people are comfortable with having intercourse while menstruating, and in my case this put a nine-month damper on my sex life. Then, after the hysterectomy, I was so sore and numb—to the point where my lower abdominal and pubic bone area didn't feel like it was a part of my body at all. Chemo also took a toll on my vagina, causing shrinking and dryness. I used vaginal cream, estrogen, lubricants and lotions. But I had to be really careful, because it's possible to tear and really hurt oneself, which ends up taking the mood away. My advice is to take it slow, and get into it only once you get comfortable.

If you had a pregnancy that was terminated because it was found to be molar, or if you miscarried, you may be experiencing a profound sense of loss or grief. These feeling can also lead to a loss of sexual desire.

Some doctors are reluctant to discuss sexual matters with their patients, unless the patients themselves bring them up. Many patients are reluctant to raise the issue with their doctors as well. As a result they don't know what to expect sexually after treatment, and they often simply suffer in silence. Obviously it's helpful in this case to have a doctor with whom you can talk openly about sexuality.

Partners may also find it difficult to initiate sex. Partners may worry that they'll be seen as selfish or not understanding of their wife's pain if they come on to her. Or they may assume she wants sex before she's ready, and may inadvertently pressure her with this assumption. Some partners find they can't cope with the physical differences caused by treatment, and they may be reluctant to restart a sexual relationship. Some partners are afraid of hurting their partner, or of catching the disease (though GTN is *not* contagious).

When I was being treated, I was so under the weather that sex was definitely not on the "to do" list. I know that nobody likes to have sex or be intimate when they have the flu. Well, imagine this being an ongoing flu that gets better, then worse again. When I have the flu, I'm not cuddly, nor am I up for sex. I don't want anyone to touch or to baby me. I also get really irritated, but I'm *not* whiny. My husband TJ is the absolute opposite. (We often joke about how it's a good thing I was the one who got sick because I wouldn't have been able to handle his whining!). Anyway, if a few months pass with no major signs of affection and there doesn't seem to be a light at the end of the tunnel, partners may feel that they're unwanted or that they're failing the relationship. This just isn't the case. It will get better; you just have to give it time. Remember: if you can get through this, you can get through anything.

Many GTN patients are eager to resume their sex-lives. But the rule is to do it because you want it, and not because of pressure from a partner. If you're feeling too tired or just aren't in the mood, don't force yourself, because you'll probably end up feeling resentful.

If you feel ready for sex, by all means go ahead. A good sex life enhances health and vitality, and the exercise might help with some of the side effects. It's important to use a reliable method of birth control, however, since pregnancy isn't recommended during treatment, or for a year following treatment. Pregnancy makes it difficult for your doctor to monitor you hCG levels (see pages 209–211 for more information on pregnancy after choriocarcinoma).

If you're having difficulty communicating with your partner about sex, you may want to try seeing a counselor. A good book whose aim is to help couples communicate about sex may also be of use. I suggest *Hot Monogamy: Essential Steps to More Passionate, Intimate Lovemaking* by Patricia Love, M.D. and Jo Robinson. This book helps couples express their needs in an open and non-judgmental manner. It's beneficial to all couples, even those who feel they have a good relationship.

When You Don't Feel Sexual But Your Partner Does

Even the most caring and sensitive partner won't be able to make up for the fact that you feel unattractive or exhausted. Furthermore, if you're experiencing temporary menopause (see pages 141–144), you may notice real physical changes (such as vaginal dryness, loss of libido due to hormonal changes, and depression) that may partly be caused by a loss of estrogen. So there may naturally be times when you're not interested in sex, but your partner is very interested.

Expanding the sexual experience is an important step when dealing with differences in levels of desire. Sex doesn't have to equal intercourse all of the time. Experiment with sensual massage, holding, hugging, masturbating your partner, or mutual masturbation. These can substitute for intercourse until you feel ready. And if vaginal dryness is the problem, you may want to try an estrogen cream.

I found that for the most part, I didn't want to be touched. I hurt all over (body aches, as I call them) and I felt nauseous—so any movement on TJ's part would start my stomach rolling. He'd get upset about this. Now that I look back on it I realize that he just wanted the cuddles and for me to show affection. I wish I'd understood that these little things (like showing affection) mean a lot, rather than being so focused on how I felt at a given moment.

TJ said: "It never seemed to matter how hard I tried: I always got shot down. I could understand that when she wasn't feeling well she wouldn't be in the mood for sex but when she wasn't feeling that bad I thought: *maybe this time it will work.* (Although she's really tough and doesn't show it very much when she's not feeling well.) When it's a fight just to get to cuddle at night you can only be told: "just don't touch me" so many times before you quit trying. It helped when we finally talked about it and just decided that if she was up for it she'd better jump me. I was tired of being turned down, and wasn't going to try to initiate anything anymore, but I was still more then willing to do it if she was in the mood."

When Both Partners Avoid Intimacy

Reestablishing sexual contact after a period of abstinence can be difficult. Many couples acknowledge that avoiding intimacy is one of the tricks they use to avoid the pain of "making the first move." This is particularly true once the ill partner is back in commission again. Either the ill partner busies herself with all the little things she needs to catch up on (so that she's exhausted by the time she goes to bed) or the well partner is so relieved that his wife is better, he wants to forget about the GTN and never discuss it again. This interferes with the couple's intimacy.

I remember when TJ and I talked about him always making the first move, and how I was always turning him down. He decided to stop and let me make the first move if and when I was in the mood, and up for sex. I'd wondered why he stopped, because I liked it when he tried—it made me feel wanted still. Just talking about it together helped us deal with some of these issues.

Tips for Reestablishing Contact
- Spend more "slowed down" time together. Go to bed earlier or stay longer in bed. Take walks together or go on a date.
- If your partner is avoiding you, let him or her know that s/he is missed. Don't lay guilt trips or blame, just express the desire to spend time together.
- Be romantic with each other. Have a second honeymoon. Courtship is an important part of reestablishing intimacy.
- Check in with each other about how you're feeling. Both partners should check on each other's emotions and health.
- Express gratitude. Think of the positive things that you've done for each other and forgive the bad.

Adapted from Dr. M. Sara Rosenthal's The Breast Sourcebook *(Lowell House: 1997).*

When You Both Feel Sexual
Sex during chemotherapy can be very beneficial, if you feel up to it. Sexually active women have fewer vaginal complications while they're receiving radiation therapy. This is because radiotherapy in the pelvic region can cause scarring in the vagina. Frequent intercourse (three to four times a week is recommended) can help separate the vaginal walls so that scar tissue doesn't form across them, closing the entrance to the vagina. You can also benefit from using a dildo or a dilator that your physician can give to you to insert into your vagina instead of intercourse. And you can try doing Kegel exercises to restore muscle strength in your vagina.

The chemo shrinking my vagina actually gave TJ even more pleasure! (Though our sex life was mostly a downer when I was sick, wasn't it honey?)

TJ says: "What can I say except take it *whenever* you can get it. It might not happen often, but when it does take advantage of it."

When a Spouse Leaves

From time to time a couple finds that they just can't weather cancer therapy together. The relationship may be causing more stress than satisfaction. In this situation, one partner may leave. Unfortunately it's usually the cancer patient who's left at a time when she most needs support. Some partners simply can't bear to watch their loved ones suffer. Though they know they shouldn't leave, they simply don't have the emotional resources to deal with everything that's going on. Some husbands leave when their wife becomes sick, then return when she's regained her health. Some couples continue this pattern throughout the duration of treatment.

Other spouses decide to leave once and for all. Spouses who don't "take you in sickness" probably weren't all that supportive when you were in health. GTN doesn't cause a spouse to leave; rather, it exposes a relationship for what it truly is. Some women who lost partners this way say that it was a curious blessing, and that they're glad they found out what kind of person their lover really was.

Finding a counselor to help you through your feelings of loss and inadequacy is imperative in this situation. It's difficult to deal with a separation or divorce in the best of circumstances, and if you're going through GTN therapy, you shouldn't try to deal with it alone.

Here is what one woman said about losing her partner after chorio:

> "My husband couldn't cope with it. He and I separated in 1979. He remains in denial today. He was very jealous of the attention I received, and accused me of acting to get everyone's attention. He told me a couple of years ago that I had "no idea what he was going through." Maybe I didn't, but I just knew that I was doing whatever I had to do to be there for him and our sons. And I thought he'd appreciate what I was going through." (Diagnosed at 27 in 1973; treated in Southampton, NY, and New York City, NY.)

FOR YOUR HUSBANDS AND PARTNERS

Up until now this book has addressed the concerns of any woman dealing with a diagnosis of GTN or choriocarcinoma. This section is aimed at her husband, spouse or partner.

First, I'd like to set aside any worries you, her partner, may have about your own chances of developing GTN. No form of GTN is contagious. Choriocarcinoma comes from a combination of your genes and your wife's genes, so you may be wondering whether you're at risk for developing cancer as well. If you've done some research you may have discovered that there exists a type of choriocarcinoma found in the testicles. This is a very different form of the cancer. Studies have shown that the male partner of a woman with choriocarcinoma is no more likely to get any form of cancer than any other male in the population. You are *not* at higher risk of developing cancer because your wife has choriocarcinoma. Furthermore, you can't catch GTN or choriocarcinoma, not even through intimate contact.

Once your wife is diagnosed with a life-threatening disease, everything changes. It may seem like all of your plans and dreams have been put on hold, at least until treatment is over. This in itself is a frustrating situation. Then there's the added uncertainty about how long treatment will last. If only the doctors could give you a definite date; at least then you could start planning for that day. However, in GTN therapy there are seldom guarantees. Even if you *are* given a time frame, you may find that this changes over the course of treatment. You may feel like you'll never be able to make plans again. TJ says: "We started treatment with the understanding that it would last about eight weeks. Well, after 10 weeks, then 20, 40, and 60 weeks, any and all plans we may have had had been passed over. Some temporarily, like Tara finishing school, and some permanently, like our having more kids. You just have to deal with each day as it comes because it's impossible to tell how long it will be before your lives return to normal."

Some spouses feel cut off from their wives because of the GTN experience. This is especially true if the husband is unable to attend many of her doctor's appointments. He'll want to know about (and understand) the latest developments in her treatment, but she may not want to go over the information again in detail. She may feel overwhelmed by the experience, and unable to really communicate what the doctor has told her. If you are able to go to her doctor's appointments, it's a good idea to do so; that way you'll be included.

Many spouses are a great source of strength during GTN treatment. Couples often surprise each other with small and caring acts. TJ was there for me as much as he could be. He'd work all night, arrive home at five in the morning, and then take me to my doctor's appointments, chemo, and so on. These appointments tended to start at around eight in the morning, and with Toronto traffic what it is at that hour, TJ had little time to sleep. He'd be by my side everywhere I had to go, and take time off work when I wanted him there—or when I was put in the hospital, because he didn't want a reoccurrence of what happened after my first treatment, with him almost losing me.

When I started losing my hair, I decided to shave it off, since I hated having to wash my pillowcase every day. TJ took me to the hairdressers and had his head shaved first, because he didn't want me to feel out of place. He looked so cute! He has this cone-head, which is pointed off-center. By the time I'd lost most of my hair, he'd shaved his own a couple of times, and I told him that I wanted him to grow it out again. He was so excited!

TJ would also make me things to eat when I was hungry, and give me my Neupogen® shots (because I couldn't handle administering them myself). He got so he was used to sleeping on hospital floors, though of course he never really got much sleep. He also put up with my whining and my bitching, and the emotional roller coaster I was on at all times. I think this must have been really hard on him.

TJ says; "It took a while but I finally realized that there was nothing I could do to fix this. Which wasn't an easy thing to accept because I'd always been able to fix things. Knowing that there was nothing I could do to make things better helped me focus on doing what little things I could to make things more comfortable and easier for Tara."

Some of the women we spoke with had this to say about the helpful things their husbands did for them during the course of their illness:

> "He read everything he could find on chorio and was very involved in my treatment. He knew how I needed to deal with things and was around when I needed him and was quiet when I didn't." (Diagnosed at 33 in 2000; treated in Toronto, Canada.)

> "I asked my husband [what he did] and he said he rubbed my back a lot! Also, he said (and it's true) that he left me alone when I needed it, and joked with me when it helped me relax." (Diagnosed at 41 in 1999; treated in Memphis, TN, then Fort Lauderdale, FL.)

> "He was there. He cried with me right after he got home, but then it was: okay, let's get down to business. He bought a calendar, kept track of things, etc." (Diagnosed in 2001; treated in Minnesota.)

Sometimes our lovers unintentionally do things that aren't helpful, or are even hurtful. Keep in mind that this situation is difficult for couples, so we're all bound to make mistakes. All the more so because GTN touches on so many different aspects of family life. TJ really wouldn't talk about how he was doing, how he was feeling and what he thought would happen if the worst (death) occurred. This upset me. I wanted to hear from him how he was dealing with everything; I certainly wanted him to "let it out."

The women we interviewed had this to say about what their husbands did that was hurtful during their treatment:

> "He had problems getting along with my family and I found that hurtful." (Diagnosed at 41 in 2002; treated in Pensacola, FL.)

> "There were a couple of days I simply *could not* get out of bed, yet I had to take care of our baby. I wanted him to stay home, but he wouldn't. Since I wasn't working, he was the sole breadwinner. I ended up asking my older daughter to stay home from school to help out." (Diagnosed in 2001; treated in Minnesota.)

> "My husband was in such denial that the day I came home from the hospital he declared: "I need laundry done you know!" I don't think my husband ever did fully cope with it himself. He kept saying: "Everything is going to be fine." I kept saying: "I have cancer." And he refused to believe it until a doctor finally spoke to him. He was in denial for a long time, so I had no help coping with the diagnosis. I was left alone to cope with it myself." (Diagnosed at 27 in 1973; treated in Southampton, NY, and New York City, NY.)

Husbands often report emotional side effects that are similar to those a patient might experience. They feel anxiety, stress and depression. They are seldom aware, however, that these are *normal* reactions. Support people tend not to share their emotional reactions to a GTN diagnosis and treatment because they feel the need to remain strong. They offer help, but they don't ask for help in return. Being a support person can be both painful and profoundly redeeming. If you're in this position, remember that it's important to care for yourself as well as your wife or partner. If you don't take care of your own needs and emotions you may find yourself burning out.

TJ says: "I kept getting yelled at for not showing any emotion, but from my point of view I wasn't allowed to because I had to be there for Tara when she was feeling bad. I had to stay strong. I burned out really quickly by doing this, but I was convinced it was the way I was supposed to act."

Here is how the women we spoke with said their husbands coped while on the chorio roller coaster:

> "He was very supportive throughout. When I finished chemo finally, he dove back into his job, and his mother moved down here, so that was hard…[His advice for other husbands going through the same thing is:] "Be there for your babe and tell her you love her all the time, even when she's bald!"… He learned about the disease along with me and I always told him my lab results, etc." (Diagnosed at 41 in 1999; treated in Memphis, TN, then Fort Lauderdale, FL.).

> "[My husband] cried after I first told him, but then was very strong throughout, which I needed *desperately!* Then, a couple months after treatment ended, he just blew! I let him release, let him yell, scream, say whatever—knowing that it was his turn to let go. Then he was his usual normal self again. [He coped by doing] research!" (Diagnosed in 2001; treated in Minnesota.)

For Husbands and Partners: Some Potential Stressors

- Feeling the need to be available 24 hours a day, 7 days a week.
- Fear of leaving your wife at home alone.
- Disruption of household routines.
- The need to change plans at the last minute.
- Balancing work outside the home with caring for your wife.
- Strained relationships with other family members. If they're involved in care you may think that they're around too much, and this may feel intrusive (which is especially true for young couples who are trying to begin a life on their own). If family members aren't involved in care, then you may feel resentment over the fact that they don't appear to want to help out.
- Feeling that you lack knowledge and/or the ability to manage your wife's physical symptoms correctly.
- Feeling inadequate as a source of emotional support to your wife (this

includes not feeling like you "know" your wife's psychological needs).

- Feeling like you lack time for yourself, time to develop and maintain supportive social relationships. Feelings of isolation.
- Concern about your own health and what would happen if you fell ill as well.
- Sleeplessness. You may wake up and feel scared about the GTN, then have difficulty getting back to sleep.
- Separation anxiety. You may feel a tremendous need to spend more time with your partner, and you may miss her more than usual when she's away. This is a normal reaction to a life-threatening illness.
- You may not want to talk about your feelings. This is a common experience for all caregivers, but particularly for male caregivers. Our culture teaches men to deal with their feelings by burying them, but that won't help here. Consider joining a support group for a safe place to talk.
- Feeling that your wife is wallowing in her GTN. Women learn to deal with their emotions by expressing them. Your wife may want to talk about the same details of her disease and her emotions over and over again. You may feel as though it isn't necessary to keep discussing the disease or its treatment, but it's by *constantly* discussing it that many women integrate the experience. If a woman wants to open up and talk, it's a sign she feels close enough to you to share.
- Feeling left out. Friends and family will frequently call to see how the ill partner's doing, but will often completely ignore her spouse's feelings. As a result you may feel scorned, resentful and/or unappreciated for all that you're doing.
- Different feelings towards sex. Since GTN and choriocarcinoma affect your wife's sex organs, you may be afraid of hurting her. She may seem more delicate in her weakened state. Or, you may not be feeling aroused because you're so tired from all the extra work you've been doing.

Adapted from: Deitra Lowdermilk and Barbara Germino "Helping Women and Their Families Cope with the Impact of Gynecologic Cancer." JOGNN: Journal of Obstetric, Gynecologic and Neonatal Nursing 29(6): 653-660, November/December 2000; *and from Dr. M. Sara Rosenthal's* The Breast Sourcebook *(Lowell House: 1997).*

There are two types of support situations: short and long term. Short-term support is much easier. It lasts anywhere from a week to a few months at most. Although there will invariably be difficulties in this type of scenario, things do get better, and perhaps this is why support people often report feeling a good deal of inner satisfaction, as well as outer gratitude (from the one they're caring for).

Long-term support is quite different. It lasts several months to several years, which means that there may be no clear end in sight. Once your extra help becomes routine, you may find that your wife no longer offers you much gratitude. As a support person, you may find that you get no rest. You may feel that no matter how many problems you have, they pale in comparison to the problems of your wife, who has cancer. So you may simply stop talking about your problems. You don't want to burden or upset you partner, because she's ill.

Your problems may well pale next to those of your wife, but knowing this doesn't make them go away. Your problems are still real problems. TJ says: "This explains exactly how I felt. My wife was 'dying'—so how could any of my problems compare to that? Naturally you end up keeping it all to yourself."

If you decide you want to talk about your feelings, the question is to whom? Support groups for caregivers are a great place to turn. Many people find that their friends can't handle all the talking that's necessary. People want to make themselves useful. Friends may not want to talk about a chronic problem because it makes them feel helpless. Support groups allow you to vent frustrations, or talk about your feelings and problems without attempting to "solve" them. In support groups for caregivers, people are allowed the space to say things they wouldn't normally. Things come out like: "Who does she think she is to order me around like that?" Or: "What makes her think she's so special just because she's sick? I've got problems of my own." Or: "I feel like I've lost control of my life." Members of the support group will understand, and see the love beneath the anger in these statements.

Support groups can also be a source of ideas about how to cope when your wife is going through chemotherapy. Caring for an ill partner is emotionally and physically draining. The longer treatment lasts, the more difficult it becomes to keep up your own energy. Watching a loved one who is unwell and in pain is frustrating, especially when there's little you can do to help.

Husbands and partners have described the strength it takes to just be there, to listen to their wives' fears and worries without trying to make them better. Some say that what they invariably become is an "emotional sponge." This is very difficult.

Male caregivers in our society often get little encouragement and support. Yet many husbands admit that meeting other men in their situation helped enormously. And many support group members end up wishing that they'd joined sooner, since they feel this would have avoided a great deal of marital or familial tension.

Tips on "Helping" for Husbands and Partners

- Go to appointments to "help" your wife listen to the information the doctor is giving her. Help make treatment decisions, but leave the final choice to her (unless she's already asked you to take on a decision-making role).
- Ask your own questions of the doctor also.
- Help in whatever ways you're good at. Try to keep the couple (or the family) focused on helping each other.
- Make the days of your appointments "date" days. You'll likely already have arranged for time off and childcare, so why not go out for lunch or to a matinee together? It's important to set aside time together that doesn't revolve around the GTN and its treatment.
- Become the homemaker without being asked. Do as much as you can around the house. Often sick people have a hard time asking for help, and yet they worry that they can't get everything done. If you take the initiative, she won't have to ask.
- Don't forget about romance. Take the day off to go on an outing. Plan a romantic weekend away. Buy her a rose or other small gift for each treatment that she makes it through. Do small things to let her know that you still love her and that you want to be with her.
- Go to a support group. Do this early so that problems don't build up and become unmanageable before you seek help. You can go to a support group for caregivers, which will give you an opportunity to vent your frustrations. Or you can go to a support group for couples, so that you'll know what other people are going through, and how they're dealing with it.

- Make her laugh. You know how to make your wife laugh better than anyone else. Bring home a funny video that you know she'll enjoy. It's important to let her know that you want to cheer her up.
- Ask her how she's feeling today. Let her know how you're feeling. GTN is an emotional experience and these emotions change from one day to the next. Consider staying in bed for an extra fifteen minutes each morning to hold each other and talk.
- Let her set the pace, depending on how she's feeling.
- Support her if she wants to talk about her GTN with your friends. People have different ways of coping, and some choose to be more open than others. Don't feel that you have to hide the fact that there is GTN in your house.

Adapted from Dr. M. Sara Rosenthal's The Breast Sourcebook *(Lowell House: 1997).*

TJ's Story

It all started with a trip to the hospital because Tara was bleeding a lot a few months after having the baby. That led to numerous trips to the doctor and a good deal of running around. When we finally got called back in to the doctor's office and were told that she had a rare type of cancer, it never really registered. Not even after being told that we needed to go to the cancer center the next day to see a specialist. I remember thinking: "It can't be that bad—she'll be in and out in no time." The doctor at the cancer center treated us like children, and because he never really told us anything, I figured it was nothing big.

We were given the run around the day of Tara's first chemo session, and when everything was finally figured out we went to the hospital for inpatient treatment. I'd worked all through the night before and then had to drive the kids to school. When I got home Tara called and told me to get back to the hospital because she wasn't feeling very well. Given the morning rush hour, it took me a while to get over there, and when I arrived Tara was gone. The nurses told me that she'd just gone down for an ultrasound, and not to worry—she'd be right back.

I was really tired from having worked all night, so the nurses suggested I sleep in Tara's hospital bed. I couldn't sleep but I did lie down, and more than two hours went by. I asked several times where Tara was but nobody could tell me. Finally our social worker came to get me. She told me that I needed to get to the ER *immediately* to sign a consent form for emergency surgery. When I finally got down there to see Tara, she looked horrible. White as a ghost, and in pain. All she could say was that she wanted it to stop hurting.

She went off to surgery, and I lost it. I completely melted down. It was the first time I really realized that this wasn't something I should be taking lightly, and that it really was serious. The social worker took Tatum from me, and suggested I find someone to come get her. I called my mother to let her know what was going on. Not that she could really understand what I was saying, but I got the point across that she'd better be on the next plane to Toronto if she ever wanted to see Tara again—because I didn't know if she'd make it out of surgery alive. Then I called Tara's parents, and with a little less "alarm" in my voice I told them to get down as soon as they could. Finally, I got in touch with one of our friends, and she said she'd leave work to come down and get the kids. I also called work, and had my boss cover my shift for me (because I was going to be at the hospital and didn't know when I'd be back). She was very understanding, and just told me to make sure I let her know when I'd be able to return to work.

Several hours and about 30 cups of coffee later, Tara finally came out of surgery. She was on morphine so she wasn't really making any sense, but she had some color back in her, and she was still alive. By the time both of our parents showed up, she was awake, drugged up, and feeling better. I received instructions from everybody to go home and get some sleep, so I unwillingly did just that.

With everyone at the hospital I was "allowed" very little time with Tara. The rest of my day was spent at work or at home sleeping. Somebody was always with the kids and somebody was always with Tara in the hospital. Things didn't really get any better when she got home. By this point I felt totally useless. I always went to chemo with Tara, but other than that we had somebody else doing *everything*: caring for *my* children, taking care of *my* house, looking after the needs of *my* wife, and so on. I was repeatedly told just to work and to rest.

And there was nothing I could do to make my wife feel any better. Not to mention the fact that she wasn't feeling well because of the chemo, so when we did interact we often fought. She felt irritable and I felt useless.

We started treatment with the understanding that Tara would have just eight weeks of chemo. A few doctors later, things started to become clear. More than a year later Tara was still going thorough chemo, and we'd had several close calls, not to mention multiple hospitalizations (because of one infection or another). I was working nights and getting what sleep I could on hospital floors. It was one of the most emotionally draining experiences I've ever had. For more than a year I spent 99 percent of my time answering the question: "How's Tara doing?" Rarely did anybody think to ask how *I* was doing. Nobody seemed to realize that having the person I love more than anything almost die on me was hard. When people did ask, it really didn't seem like I was allowed to say anything, because she was the one who was sick.

Well, chemo is over now and Tara's feeling better. We're talking again, and working out the problems that arose in our relationship as a result of her being sick. It wasn't easy, but I'm glad we made it through this. We're stronger than ever now.

CHILDREN

A study of adult patients with a variety of cancers found that a full 24 percent were parenting children throughout the course of their treatment. Although no such study has looked specifically at GTN or choriocarcinoma, it's reasonable to assume that the percentage would be much higher, since this group of diseases affects women who are young and still in their childbearing years. We know that many patients have kids; however, there have been very few studies that look at how these patients (and parents) are managing childcare while they recover. Furthermore, there are very few studies that look at how the children of patients cope with their parent's illness.

The parents we spoke with had this to say about coping with parenting during treatment:

> "[I coped with parenting] the best I could! [I] tried to keep their home life as normal as possible. [My daughter] had a few days when she claimed she was too sick to go to school. [My husband] brought her to the hospital to stay with me. She wasn't sick; she just wanted to be with me. She usually slept in the bed with me, and she loved getting a snow cone while she was there! The nurses and doctors were very good about it." (Diagnosed in 2001; treated in Minnesota.)

> "If the children are old enough to help you, get them involved. It

makes them feel good about themselves and the fact that they can help mommy. Depending upon their age, divide chores up for them to do: [they can] dust, take out the garbage, give themselves a bath, etc. Even a four year-old can dust!" (Diagnosed at 27 in 1973; treated in Southampton, NY, and New York City, NY.)

Children Can Be a Source of Joy and Strength

The pride and pleasure that most parents feel in their children is often a welcome departure from the sadness, anger and anxiety that sometimes accompanies GTN treatment. When you're feeling down in the dumps, a kind gesture from your child might be enough to lift you back up. Just watching both my kids helped me through this—Tragean and Tatum playing, making each other laugh. Tatum learning new things and Tragean teaching them to her was so delightful, a real pleasure to watch. Although I couldn't be there for them in the way I would have liked, getting better was my main priority. I knew that if I were able to pull through this, I'd be able to spend a whole bunch of time with them later.

Here's what the parents we spoke with said about their children (and, in one case, their cat!) helping:

"Actually, I think [my kids] were my best medicine. Just having them around helped me cope with everything." (Diagnosed at 27 in 1973; treated in Southampton, NY, and New York City, NY.)

"At diagnosis [my children were] 19, 17, and 9, plus our newborn. [The older girls] helped with baby, and took care of themselves for the most part when I could not." (Diagnosed in 2001; treated in Minnesota.)

"Pets are a great comfort for someone who is at home alone. My cat never left my side and would spend her days beside me on the couch. This was a great comfort, since I didn't have any children." (Diagnosed at 33 in 2000; treated in Toronto, Canada.)

Helping Children Cope

Children do best with a regular schedule and should be encouraged to continue with their life "as usual." For very young children this means maintaining regular sleeping and eating times. For older children this is also a concern, as is sticking to regular school, social and extra-curricular activities and schedules. This won't always be easy, since your own schedule will have to be adjusted to accommodate your treatments and periods of rest. But try to settle into a new routine if possible. Inform your child's caretakers (baby-sitters, teachers, administrators, etc.) about the state of your health and its impact on your family. This will allow your child's support network to be accommodating to your child's needs. If making all these phone calls is too difficult, consider asking the mother of your child's best-friend to do it for you. When family life is disrupted by illness, stability in other areas of a child's life is especially important.

You should also encourage your child to form relationships with non-parental adults, such as the parents of their friends or your own friends. It helps children to have an adult outside of the family unit with whom they can discuss their fears. Just like adults, children sometimes feel that they should be strong—and not express their fears to their parents. You can say things like: "It makes me feel good to hear that you and [non-parental adult] figured that out together." This sends the message that the child's other relationships with adults are appreciated and not seen as disloyal to you.

Tragean and Tatum bonded with everyone that came to help out. Both kids were really good with dealing with change—Tragean more so than Tatum since he was able to better understand what was happening, and to ask questions.

It's easiest to accommodate an illness in the family when both parents work well together and relate well to their children. If the relationship between you and your husband is strong, you're less likely to fear for your child's future in the event that something should happen to you. However, if there's preexisting parental discord, or if you're divorced, creating a support network for your child might be more difficult. Some divorced parents (or single moms) can work things out alone, while others rely on extended family members to bridge the gap. Often, however, professionals are required. If you find you can't communicate with the father of your children, it might be a good idea to enlist the services of a mediator. Mediators can suggest ways to create routine that will be in the best interests of the child.

Tragean's Story

We interviewed my son to get a sense of how children cope with having a parent with choriocarcinoma. Here's what he said:

Q: *How did you feel when you first found out?*

A: I felt pretty sad, and I thought that you were going to die. Then you gave me the teddy bear and I felt a lot better. I slept with it every night. I always asked if you were going to die and you always told me that if you had your way you weren't going to die, and that you always had your way.

Q: *What were you thinking the first time you went to the hospital?*

A: I was thinking that you were going to be okay. And then I was scared because I kept on having bad dreams and stuff about you dying and then having to bury you. The nurses and the doctors were nice. It was a little bit boring there, because there was nothing to do, until I found out there was a TV in another room.

Q: *What were your thoughts on me sleeping all the time?*

A: It was pretty boring because we used to have fun (and we still do now). We played football together and went in the sprinkler together and it was fun.

Q: *Did you like having people stay with us?*

A: Yes, it made me feel a little bit better.

Q: *How was school when I was sick?*

A: It was pretty good except for the kids that made fun of me.

Q: *How did they make fun of you?*

A: They said things like "you're mom's bald!" and stuff like that.

Q: *Were the teachers nice?*

A: Yeah. They told the kids that they had detention because they weren't supposed to make fun of people who have cancer. And then the kids in my class didn't make fun of me anymore. They would start helping me at recess when kids from other classes would bug me.

Q: *Anything else you'd like to add? Any advice to other kids going through this?*

A: Even if your mom has cancer, don't worry because she might get her way and not die. That's my advice. But you might go through some pretty hard things.

Talking with Children about GTN

Some parents don't want to discuss illness with their children. They don't want to burden their children with such a heavy subject. However, children are very perceptive. They tend to notice when something's wrong. If you don't keep your child informed, he or she may feel uncertain and scared. Open communication reassures your child that the family will get through the illness, regardless of outcome. It also lets your child know that you'll weather the uncertainty together. Furthermore, the extra time spent cuddling and talking with your child will assure him or her that he or she isn't the cause of the disruption, and is still loved.

Explaining things in an age-appropriate manner is key to promoting a child's understanding. However, it's important to remember that each child develops at a different rate. Our guidelines for talking to children about illness are listed according to age, but you know your child best. If you feel that using an "older" or "younger" approach is more appropriate in the case of your child, by all means do so.

Ages 3–7

Children in this age group weave together logic and fantasy to arrive at their own, very unique understanding of events in the world. They're often egocentric, and cast themselves at the center (or as the cause) of events that are affecting them. Because of this, it's important to remind children of this age that the illness is not the result of anything they did or thought. You can say things like: "Some kids worry that they somehow caused the cancer, but this is never true." You can also ask your child what he or she thinks caused the cancer, so that any misconceptions can be dispelled.

Signs that your child may be feeling distressed about your illness are anxious or inhibited behavior, or outbursts of angry, oppositional behavior. I really can't remember Tragean acting any differently, other than when the kids in school were making fun of the fact that I'd lost my hair, and telling him that he had my germs. We've only had that problem since we moved back to Saskatchewan. The school in Toronto was absolutely amazing, and took extra time to help make him feel better. He told his friends that I had cancer like it was something to be proud of! Maybe it made him feel like he was smarter than them, or like he had access to a world they didn't—who knows?

181

Ages 7–12

Children in this age group have a more realistic worldview, yet they may still feel guilty about things that they've said or done. Educating them about GTN can help them to understand that their behavior did nothing to cause it. You might also let children in this age group know that GTN is not contagious. Children in this age group do understand the permanence of death, so the possibility of death as an outcome may be a part of your discussions (see pages 205–207) for more information on talking with children about death).

Children sometimes ask questions in roundabout ways. You can facilitate communication by welcoming their curiosity, and taking the time to explore the "real" questions behind it. Saying things like: "What got you wondering about that?" or "What part did you want to know about?" will help to draw out your child's underlying concern.

You don't need to feel that you should have all the answers. It's possible to receive each question warmly, even if you don't know how to address it. You can say things like: "That's an important question. Let me think about it." But do remember to revisit it once you've had time to formulate a response. You might also say: "I'd like to talk about it with Daddy (or the doctor) before answering." Again, it should be you who raises it the second time; that way, your child will know that the question is important to you, regardless of whether or not you know how to answer it.

Misinformation from others is difficult to avoid. Well-meaning people will say things to and around your child that are neither accurate nor helpful. For example, your child might hear frightening stories about other people's experience with cancer, which may not be relevant your situation with choriocarcinoma or GTN. You should encourage your child to share these stories with you, so that you can correct any misinformation.

Teenagers

By the time they've reached their teen years, your kids will have developed a logical understanding of the world and will be able to understand the implications of a GTN diagnosis. However, the teenage years are a time when children are seeking independence, and trying to define themselves as unique and separate from their parents. A seriously ill parent may interfere with this developmental step. Some adolescents become more dependent on or attached to the sick parent. Some experience no difficulty at all in adjusting, while others rebel.

Adolescents may experience a wide range of reactions to a parent's diagnosis. They may want to help as much as possible. Or, they may resent the extra chores and the time these chores take away from activities that they enjoy. They may feel angry and guilty about wanting to flee. This reaction can be especially difficult for your teenager if the two of you weren't getting along very well before the illness.

Older adolescents may feel overwhelmed by the parent's pain and by their own helplessness in dealing with it. As a result, they may become aloof. Others may become anxiously over-involved in the parent's care. And still others may act out aggressively and destructively (they may turn to alcohol and drugs, or get into fights) or may abandon their social outlets entirely.

Some teens may begin to fail in school. Some may even start developing headaches, rashes, and other psychosomatic problems. Finally, teens that are particularly mature may cope as adults do, seeking and evaluating information and turning to friends and counselors for help.

Teens are aware of cancer news in the media. If you have a teenage daughter, she may have heard that some cancers are inheritable, and she may be worried that the same thing might happen to her. You can assure her that there's no evidence that either GTN or choriocarcinoma runs in families. It is not an inherited disease.

Some Common Question Parents Have about Discussing GTN or Choriocarcinoma with Children

- *"What should we call the illness?"* Just call it what it is (a mole, or choriocarcinoma; or you could refer to it as cancer), though you may have to explain what this means. If you use euphemisms like "boo-boo," your child may get confused and think that any hurt can become a serious illness.
- *"How much should we share with our children?"* Parents often want to protect their children from bad news. However, children are remarkable in their ability to pay attention to adult conversation, even when they don't appear to be listening. You should assume that anything you're discussing will be heard by your children. Trying to protect them may actually be more harmful than addressing the situation. Openly discussing the situation conveys the message that you don't want your child to worry alone.

- *"When should I talk to my child about the illness?"* It's important to choose a time when both parents are feeling calm. If you live in a two-parent household, both parents should talk to the children together. Single parents might want to ask a good friend or relative to help them through the conversation.

- *"Should I make my child talk about my illness?"* Once you've made it clear to your child that you're available to talk and that you're interested in your child's thoughts and worries, it's usually best to let the child initiate discussions. On the other hand, if your child never discusses the illness you may want to make an unintrusive comment such as: "You know that if you want to talk about the GTN (mole or choriocarcinoma) I'd be interested in what it was like for you." But don't push it.

- *"Are there typical reactions that I should look for?"* Children often don't express their reactions in words. Parents get clues about how their children are feeling by watching their behavior. If your child seems to be acting strangely or acting out, it may be his or her way of showing that he or she is upset. You might say something like: "I know everyone is worried right now, but let's find a way to talk about it rather than fighting."

- *"How will I know if my child needs help?"* The most important thing to look for is how extreme the behavioral change is and how long it's been going on. If the usual methods of handling this aren't working and the child is unable to accept extra support, professional help may be the answer. It can be useful to talk with the child's pediatrician, school counselor, or with the counseling staff at the hospital where the parent is receiving treatment.

Adapted from Paula Rauch, Anna Muriel and Ned Cassem "Parents With Cancer: Who's looking After the Children?" Journal of Clinical Oncology, 20(21): 4399-4402, November 2002.

Preparing Children for the Hospital Visit

If you are hospitalized and your child wants to visit you, it's best to accommodate your child's wishes. However, it's best to prepare your child and have another adult there to facilitate the visit if possible. There *is* one exception, and that's if you're delirious, agitated or heavily medicated, and may not recognize your child. In this case it may be best to postpone the visit until you've recovered. Young children may not understand their mother's altered state, and may be frightened by the experience.

If your child doesn't want to visit you in the hospital it's a good idea to find out why. Your child may have a specific fear that you can dispel. If it helps, you can ask hospital staff to postpone (if it's possible) any procedures until your child has left. If your child still doesn't want to go to the hospital after you've reassured him or her, then it may be best to respect his or her wishes. The exception to this of course is if you're very ill, and don't expect to return home.

If your child doesn't want to visit, offering other means of communication may be helpful. You could have the child call the hospital, draw, write letters, record tapes or videos, or write emails. Let your child know that his or her efforts at communicating please you. For example you might say: "Your drawing is right beside my bed. I smile each time I see it."

Before you take your children to the hospital, you or another trusted adult should prepare them for what they're likely to see. Discuss your appearance if it's changed (e.g., if your hair fell out during hospitalization), IV lines, oxygen masks, roommates, doctors and nurses. The visit should last as long (or as short) as your child wants. A familiar adult who will be willing to leave when the children are ready should accompany them. This can be the father, but if he wants to stay for a longer visit, then you should enlist the help of a friend. After the visit your children should be given the opportunity to discuss anything about the visit that they want to with you, their father or with another trusted adult. The adult may want to ask them which parts were fun and which parts, hard. You can also use this opportunity to discuss any additional questions that the child may have.

EXTENDED FAMILY

In a perfect world your family would focus solely on you. But everyone has an opinion about what you should be doing and how you should be dealing with your GTN diagnosis. Sometimes this can cause friction with family members who are too pushy.

Here are some tips for family members relayed to us by the women we interviewed:

"Remember: it's all about the patient. Her interest is where the emphasis should be placed." (Diagnosed at 41 in 2002; treated in Pensacola, FL.)

"Tell people not to ask what they can do, [and instead] just do it. Show up with a meal, offer to run an errand, help with laundry. I hated to ask anyone for anything as I didn't want to impose on them." (Diagnosed at 33 in 2000; treated in Toronto, Canada.)

"[My family helped by] just listening when I needed to vent, [and telling] stories of cancer patients that had a happy ending. Sometimes just hearing about what the neighbors back home were doing, etc. [really helped] to get my mind off things." (Diagnosed at 41 in 1999; treated in Memphis, TN, then Fort Lauderdale, FL.)

Family members are the most consistent sources of support and help. Whether you like it or not, you'll probably have to turn to your family for help while you're undergoing treatment for GTN or choriocarcinoma. On the other hand, family members may be too protective. Although they're probably trying to keep your interests in mind, this isn't always the case. A couple of the women we interviewed had this to say about the things their family members did that were harmful:

"[They talked] too much when I was tired and everyone wanted to come and see me in the hospital and I found that very draining." (Diagnosed at 33 in 2000; treated in Toronto, Canada.)

"[My family had] squabbles with my husband, but most of that was his lack of coping." (Diagnosed at 41 in 2002; treated in Pensacola, FL.)

Judy's Story

It seems like it was only yesterday when I received the phone call from my son Terry, or "TJ" to the rest of the world. Wayne, my hubby, and I had just spent a lovely two weeks in the Dominican and had only been back a few days when the world around us came crashing down.

I was busy working when the phone rang. It was Terry, and after some chitchat he asked me to call Tara and cheer her up. I asked why, only to hear Terry tell me that they'd just found out that Tara had cancer. The tears came then, and there was no stopping them. We spoke for a few minutes more, but what was said was a blur. I hung up the phone in shock and disbelief. These children were just starting their lives together; and they had a new baby to deal with! This didn't happen to young people—only old people, people who'd already lived their lives. A few minutes later the phone rang again. Terry had called back to advise me that I had to quit crying before I called Tara, or there was no way I'd cheer her up. At least we got a chuckle from that.

Tara and I chatted on and off over the next week and a half, learning together about her particular type of cancer and about what had to be done. On Friday, February 15, 2002, another great day at work, my concentration level was not where it was supposed to be, what with Tara constantly on my mind. I knew they were at the hospital. I left a message on Terry's phone to call and let me know how things were. The next thing I know Terry calls in such a state he's almost incomprehensible. Something had happened to Tara. My heart raced and I shook with the fear that I was about to be told the worst. Terry managed to tell me that Tara was in emergency surgery and that she was hemorrhaging profusely. He didn't actually know how she was doing. I was concerned for the children—where were they? Who was looking after them? (Tragean was in school, and the social worker was looking after Tatum.) Terry wanted me in Toronto, and I knew that I had to be there to see for myself that all was okay. But at this time, all was definitely not okay.

I called Wayne to tell him that I was going to Toronto My boss, being the understanding person he is, wasn't sure what had hit our office that morning. We'd spoken earlier (he wasn't in the office) and all had been fine. The next thing he knew I was leaving for Toronto. I'd booked a flight and was packed and at the airport within two hours. It was the longest flight of my life—not knowing if Tara was okay, and if my son had lost his wife and my grandchildren, their mother. (The mind certainly plays games when there's no one to talk with.)

When I finally walked into the hospital room, I found my son sitting beside one very sweet sight. (A quick kiss on the head for him and a very warm hug and kiss for Tara, who looked like shit.) She was white as a ghost, and yet was still smiling her usual infectious smile. The relief of knowing and seeing that all was okay, and that Tara was alive, was very overwhelming.

With everything that happened next, we seemed to forget someone very important, TJ. It was like he didn't even exist. Tara's folks arrived after midnight. Terry was told that evening to go home and get some sleep (my idea, as I was worried about him). Things needed to be done, and Terry didn't seem capable of doing any of them. He did well before we got there and just fine after we all left, but during the time the parents were around, he was incapable of anything. I don't believe it was his choice to be pushed aside; the parents just took over. And in order not to hurt anybody's feelings, TJ did as he was told.

As parents, we sometimes believe our children can't make it on their own. So, we pick them up when they're down. Groceries had to be bought, and they needed help with the kids. Just being there gave me peace of mind, as I could witness Tara's good (and bad) days.

We talked lots and lots after my return home. I needed to know that all was well. They called after every chemo treatment, and every time there was bloodwork done. I really wanted to be there, but at this point they had so much help they didn't need me hanging around. They went from living by themselves as a family to having somebody with them seven days a week. That would put a lot of stress on anybody. However, for us to offer them more support they'd need to move home, and wouldn't. These kids wanted to prove that they could survive on their own, and they also felt that the doctors were better in Toronto (they had more cases there than here in Saskatoon, as I'd find out later).

My next visit was in May, and I could hardly wait for it to come. This time I went for five days. Seeing the two of them and the kids was great. Tara was feeling rather well when I was there, as my visit feel on one of her "good" weeks. She went through chemo each week, but one week was always worse than the others. After this we still chatted lots on the phone, and I made sure that they keep me up to date on the counts and how everyone was doing. I finally agreed to come out and help in September; all I needed to know was how long they wanted me to stay. Tara asked if I could come for six weeks. This request turned out to be the turning point for the next series of events. I asked for the time off from work, but because I worked in such a small office, I wasn't able to get it without my losing my job. I told TJ and Tara that they needed to move home, or at the very least to just send the kids (I'd keep them until Tara was done her chemo and was able to look after her family again). Tara and TJ agreed to this, and I was happy to see the kids here.

After many conversations and much deliberation on Tara's part, she agreed to complete her chemo in Saskatoon. We arranged it with the Cancer Center here, and got everything in order for Tara's arrival. I took the kids to the airport to get their mom and the tears started to well as soon as I saw this very pale, fragile-looking girl come through the doors. The children were excited.

Tara was having good days and bad days with her chemo. We pulled together and did what needed to be done. And then the good news that came in April 2003 was that Tara's chemo was over. Since then, the results of her bloodwork have been good, and we thank the good lord for letting us keep her.

FRIENDS

Illness can make friendships stronger, but it can also cause friends to drift. If some of your friends disappear, this doesn't necessarily mean that they weren't good friends. Some people have a very difficult time dealing with illness, and they may find it hard to see a friend in a weakened state. Remember that there will always be others who stick by your side, becoming valuable confidants throughout the recovery process.

Telling your friends about a GTN diagnosis can be difficult. You may still be in shock yourself, and as a result your friend's questions may seem frightening. Or, you may not want to talk about your GTN at all. You may want to talk, but have no idea where to start. I had a lot of friends and family call to see how I was doing, check up on my counts, and so on. But there were many times I'd tell whoever answered to just say I was sleeping, because I really had no energy to talk, or I was sick, at that moment, of talking about cancer.

The women we interviewed had different approaches to telling their family and friends about their diagnosis:

> "I got my husband to [tell my family] and I wouldn't speak to them for weeks, even my Mum. I was just far too upset at having lost my baby and having this ridiculous disease. [As for friends] I wouldn't speak to anyone for weeks. I lost touch with my best friend because she was pregnant and was due when I would have been. I just couldn't face her and the fact that she was going to have the baby I should have been having." (Diagnosed at 30 in 1997; treated in Sheffield, UK.)

> "We were living in Memphis, with no family around, so all communication was by phone. I never told my cousins, [and] my mother

took care of passing along any news. I only told very close friends [with whom I communicated] via email while I lived in Memphis. When we moved back [here] to Florida, only two girlfriends knew about it." (Diagnosed at 41 in 1999; treated in Memphis, TN, then Fort Lauderdale, FL.)

Tips for Telling Your Friends and Relatives About GTN

- *Break the news at your own pace.* You may be feeling overwhelmed and unready to discuss the diagnosis. However, your friends and family are no doubt anxiously awaiting news of the results of your tests. This can put pressure on you to talk when you're not ready. Sometimes simply saying: "What I feared, happened" is enough to let people know.
- *Choose language that suits you.* Some people prefer not to use the words "GTN" "choriocarcinoma" or "cancer." Others prefer to say "I was diagnosed with GTN (or cancer)," rather than "I have GTN (or cancer)," as a way to disown the disease. There is no one right way to talk about your illness, so do whatever makes you feel comfortable.
- *Enlist help from others.* You can ask your friends to help you spread the news. If you don't feel like discussing the GTN over and over again you can ask a close friend or relative to take care of these details for you. That way you can save your phone conversations for the more positive topics in life.
- *Be prepared for people's curiosity.* People may ask about your treatments and about how you're feeling. They may ask you about personal details concerning your health. You don't have to answer if you don't feel comfortable. Saying: "I don't know right now," or "I'm still in too much shock to think about that," is perfectly acceptable.
- *Remember that it's okay to draw boundaries.* You don't have to answer every question that's asked. It's up to you how much you want to talk about, and how many intimate details you're interested in sharing. It's perfectly fine to make use one of the answers above, or to simply change the topic of conversation.
- *Remember that it's okay to express emotion.* If you feel sad when you're talking about the GTN, you don't have to feel shy. The situation surrounding GTN is very emotional and it isn't weak on your part to

let these emotions out sometimes. Don't ignore your own need to talk to someone. Setting up a false front, or "happy face" to disguise how you feel is not helpful to you or to your friends and family.

- *Remember that it's okay to be direct and to let people know what you need from them, even if what you need is to be left alone for a while.* However, try to avoid completely neglecting a friend or relative who wants to talk with you.

Adapted from Lorraine V. Murray "Breaking the News about Your Diagnosis" www.cancer.org/.

FOR YOUR FRIENDS

When I asked one friend who no longer came around why she'd disappeared, she said it was because she didn't know how to help, and felt useless. This situation is difficult and self-perpetuating. The only way to know how to help is to be involved. But if the friend doesn't know how to help he or she may just feel "in the way," and may be uncomfortable trying to be involved. Moreover, it often takes a while for friends to realize that chemotherapy doesn't change friendship. This is because friends often feel they should be doing something. What's important to remember is that just being a friend is doing something.

Most people (sick and healthy alike) find it difficult to ask for help. If you find yourself hanging back as a friend, or waiting to be asked for help, you may end up waiting a very long time.

Here is what the women we spoke with said was helpful from their friends:

> "Work friends behaved appallingly. Nobody phoned, wrote or anything to see how I was. All they were bothered about was the fact that they saw me in the pub on a Friday night and so couldn't work out why I wasn't going to work. Didn't ask to find out that I was due for more chemo on Monday, out on Wednesday, sick and tired Thursday, tired Friday, picked up Friday evening and ready to start all over again on Monday." (Diagnosed at 30 in 1997; treated in Sheffield, UK.)

"[My friends] drove me to chemo, came with me to appointments, held a fundraiser, brought me treats, and called me on a regular basis." (Diagnosed at 33 in 2000; treated in Toronto, Canada.)

"I think a lot of them were afraid of 'getting what I had' because they didn't really understand it, so most of them stayed away for a very long time. Today my friends stick together better. I think staying away from me like I had the 'cooties' was hurtful, but I understood. After my separation [from my husband], most of them came around." (Diagnosed at 27 in 1973; treated in Southampton, NY, and New York City, NY.)

Meredith's Story

When Tara first told me about her cancer diagnosis, the news didn't register at all. I was sitting in my office doing research for a book on gynecology when she called. She told me that she had some bad news—that she had cancer of the placenta. I said something like: "Oh, I'm sorry to hear that." Like it was nothing, a broken arm or something. We chatted for a bit and I went back to work. About ten minutes later it hit me. *Wait a minute—I think Tara just told me she has cancer!* I called her back and asked if I could come over. I don't know why it took that long for the news to register, and I felt really bad for just brushing it off at first. I arrived at Tara's with the book I was researching (*The Gynecological Sourcebook* by Dr. M. Sara Rosenthal) and we read the section on gynecological cancer. Everything seemed very confusing.

My aunt and I had planned a trip to Mexico and were scheduled to leave the day after Tara started chemotherapy. When I got back I got a call saying that something had gone wrong, and that Tara had had a hysterectomy. I went straight from the airport to Tara's house. I didn't even drop off my suitcase. When I arrived I was surprised to see how much had changed in the week that I'd been away. When I left Tara was still strong, and things at her house were still calm and orderly. When I saw Tara again, she couldn't stand straight because of the pain from her abdominal surgery. What was worse, it hurt her to laugh. Whenever I think of Tara the first thing that pops into my head is her joyous and infectious laughter. It seemed wrong to see her in pain when she laughed.

To make things even stranger, Tatum, Tara's 10 month-old daughter, was crying. Now, most people don't think it sounds strange to hear a 10 month-old cry, but before this Tatum rarely made a fuss. Tatum was teething and had been weaned suddenly when chemo started. The combination made her fussier than usual. Tara's dad was visiting from Saskatchewan in order to care for Tara and her kids, and he was trying to calm Tatum down. What could I do? I felt out of place, I didn't know what I could possibly do to help. I felt I should leave, but I didn't; I spent the night. I didn't sleep well though—and instead spent the night scolding myself for not knowing what to do. I kept thinking: *How could this happen? Tara seems so young and healthy.* It just didn't make sense. Finally, I slept.

The next morning when Tatum woke up I went to get her out of bed so that Tara and her husband (and Tara's father) could get a few extra minutes of sleep. I realized that it was normal for Tara to be in pain after surgery, and that Tara would get better (and she did, after she'd healed from the abdominal surgery). Eventually I realized that I didn't really have to do anything to help. I could just continue to be Tara's friend. In some ways things had changed, but the important thing remained the same. Tara was the same great friend that she'd always been, and we could still talk about all the same stuff.

It's true that having a friend with cancer can make you sad, and it certainly made me sad sometimes. But Tara and I make each other laugh a lot. She thinks I'm funny when we watch horror movies (I'm a chicken, and jump at everything). When Tara was hospitalized with an infection, I visited many times. If there's one thing about hospitals, it's that they're boring! We talked and visited, but there was nothing to do. Our conversation seemed forced at the hospital, like we were both obviously not talking about the fact that we were in a hospital. So the next day when I came back to visit I stuffed a sleeping bag, popcorn, TV and VCR into my bag and brought along some movies. When I showed up and started pulling the stuff out of my bag Tara laughed and laughed. We popped some popcorn in the ward microwave and had a film night sleepover.

Later, Tara and I decided to write this book. It was good to have a project we could work on together. Doing the research gave us something to do while we were waiting in the hospital for Tara's chemo treatments. I think that going through this experience together has strengthened our friendship. I know that Tara will be my friend for life and that I can count on her to be there for me if I need her. I'm not proud of the way that I acted all of the time, and sometimes I think I could have been more supportive and helpful. But when

I think about it, this is true of any friendship, whether or not cancer is a part. I've tried to forgive myself for my failings and to focus on the bond between Tara, her family, and me.

Melissa's Story

When Tara called me to tell me she'd been diagnosed with cancer, my heart did one big flip flop, and I had to remind myself to breathe. Then my brain kicked back in and I started to think a bit more rationally. I've seen many members of my family battle cancer, so I thought to myself: *If this is like cervical cancer, she has an 80 percent chance of survival. She caught it in time, and she'll be OK… she's a fighter, she'll get through.* Being in Saskatoon at the time, I felt very helpless. I wasn't there with her to reassure her, and I couldn't do anything but pray and hope for the best.

It's easy to be strong for someone when they live thousands of kilometers away, and you don't have to see them suffering. I had lots of positive things to say on the phone and by email. I imagined a healthy Tara, not a sick one. But when I got off the plane in Toronto that June and saw how much weight she'd lost, and how she had no hair anywhere, all those positive words of encouragement seemed to disappear from my lips. All I saw was how cancer had affected her body. And when we got back to her place from the airport, I felt like I was always in the way. I watched what I said so I wouldn't upset her; I tried not to be too loud so she could sleep. I walked on eggshells for the first few days of my visit. But I did relax a little when I got used to the routine.

Tara was feeling good one day so we went to Niagara Falls. For that one day, I felt like I was with the friend I remembered, Tara before she got sick. She was laughing and had loads of energy, just like she always did. I saw her with 20 extra pounds, and with her long hair. It was a good day, one I'll never forget. It was the best part of my stay. The worst part was when Tara invited me to come with her to a chemo treatment. When the medicine went in, she became as green as Kermit the Frog. She seemed to visibly get smaller.

That week was one filled with a lot of different emotions for me—excitement to see my friend, sadness and helplessness when I saw her suffering, nervousness, and finally anger that this whole thing was happening. But I don't regret going out to Toronto that week; I learned a lot and I became closer to my friend. After that, I was never nervous talking to her about cancer. I don't watch what I say anymore at all. I've accepted that Tara is sick and I'm ready to deal with whatever comes next. She's on the road to recovery now, and I truly believe that she made it this far because her family and friends insisted she keep a positive attitude. If she'd given up hope I think she'd have been gone in less than a month. So, if you have a friend or family member who is sick, remember that even though it may not seem like it at the time, your support and love really does help.

Sarah's Story

It was late when Tara phoned to tell me she had cancer. I remember being more upset than I wanted to admit. It didn't seem real, and it still doesn't. The only thing that I could think to do was to offer to tell our friends. But there was no easy or right way to tell them, and I ended up just blurting it out. It was my way of keeping my sadness hidden. I never really felt like I was entitled to my feelings. After all, I wasn't the one who was sick. I still wish I could go back and do a better job—but of course I hope I'll never get that chance.

I was surprised by the differences in our friends' reactions. They ranged from obvious emotion to the absence of it. The news hit some people hard and fast, while others needed more time to absorb what I'd told them.

I flew to Toronto for a visit about four months after the diagnosis. I didn't even recognize the person who came to pick me up at the airport. I was shocked at how pale and thin Tara looked. I spent a lot of time that week playing with the kids. Clearly they were what held everything and everyone together.

How Do I Help?

One of the things you'll learn as a support person is that you don't have to "help" so much as you have to continue to be a good friend. Many people feel helpless because nothing they can do will get rid of the GTN. But there are still many things you can do that are helpful, you just need to be considerate and look for opportunities to help as they arise rather than trying to plan the help in advance. If you're worrying about what you can do you might miss important opportunities to spend time with your friend. Just listening to your friend's concerns may be enough. Staying involved with your friend's life will give you ideas about activities that you can do together—ideas that are appropriate to your friend's health and energy level.

Tips on Helping Your Friend with GTN

- Don't ask if you can help. Just do it. Most people hate asking for help. It's probably difficult for your friend with GTN to think of what exactly needs to be done. So, think of things you appreciate when you're sick, and just do them.
- Cook some meals that can be frozen in advance, and bring them along on your next visit.
- Bring your laundry to your friend's house and do your laundry and your friend's at the same time. This way you're not taking on extra work (you'd have to do your own laundry anyway) but you are doing something to help out.
- Invite your friend's family over to your house, or on an outing. This will give your friend some time alone to rest.
- Offer to drive your friend to her chemotherapy appointments. Even if her husband usually does this, he may appreciate the break.
- Offer to babysit, or offer to take your friend's children to their appointments and extra curricular activities. If your friend has extended family staying with them to help, invite everyone out for a fun day or evening. This could give your friend and her husband a night to themselves (they may find they lack privacy, especially if they have a lot of people helping out).
- Listen to your friend if she needs to vent her frustrations with her family or her situation. And remember that you don't need to fix her problems. Your friend obviously has a lot going on, and she may just need an opportunity to verbalize her emotions without hurting anyone's feelings. Don't offer advice. Just listen.
- Act normal. Don't treat her differently because of her diagnosis. Respond to her needs, but don't pity her or the situation.
- Don't try to cheer her up if she's depressed. It's normal to be depressed when faced with a life-threatening illness, and if you try to cheer her up she may feel that you're dismissing her concerns.
- Talk about things other than her GTN. Dealing with doctors all day can make anyone feel like a set of statistics. You can remind your friend that she is a person, too. Talk about all the same things you did before the diagnosis.
- Don't judge! You may not think that your friend, her husband or her

children are dealing with the situation very well. But it isn't your place to make comments about any of it. Everyone deals with things in their own way. Remember, although you love your friend very much, the experience is fundamentally different for her family members than it is for you. Your friend may want to complain to you about her husband or children, but it's *never* okay for you to make these kinds of complaints, not even if she brings it up. Simply listen and let her say her piece.

- Be understanding and patient with your friend if she isn't acting like her old self. The drugs used in chemotherapy can affect a patient's mood and perception.

Adapted from Meredith and Tara's experience, the Canadian Cancer Society's booklet "Taking Time" and the American Cancer Society's webpage "For Spouses, Family and Friends."

How Should I Talk to My Friend with GTN?

Some people feel uncomfortable talking to people who are sick. They fear that they won't know what to say and that the long silences will make the situation awkward. But there really is no "right" way to talk to someone with a serious illness. There are no "right" things to say. The best way to deal with someone with a serious disease is to be yourself, and treat her exactly as you always have.

It's a good idea to let your friend take the lead. And definitely don't nag or judge. There are many different ways of coping with an illness, and if your friend is doing it differently than you would, that's okay. As long as her methods of coping aren't life-threatening (i.e., she's not turning to drugs or alcohol for escape) you should just let her get on with it as best as she can.

When Meredith and other friends visited, I still wanted to gab, and have a bitch session if needed. Or even just veg on the couch and watch movies. I wanted the same friendship we had before. Knowing that it was different because I was feeling different made it very hard to pick up where our friendship left off—before the diagnosis. Soon we learned the boundaries of what we could and couldn't do together anymore (like walking long distances on the lakefront), and we changed our friendship accordingly.

I'm so lucky to have the friends and family that I do. The support and everything I got from everyone was amazing. For tips on talking to your friend with cancer, see the American Cancer Society's webpage entitled: "Suggestions for Talking with the Person with Cancer" (*http://www.cancer.org/*).

CHAPTER 8

COMMON FEARS ABOUT GTN TREATMENT

LOSS OF FERTILITY

If you did not have a hysterectomy as part of your GTN therapy, then chances are good your fertility will be preserved, even if you have to undergo chemotherapy. In a small number of cases, however, chemotherapy treatment leads to chemically induced premature menopause. This condition occurs when the chemotherapy drugs affect the functioning of your ovaries. Usually these effects on the ovaries are temporary, and the ovaries return to normal functioning once chemotherapy is stopped. Sometimes, however, the damage is irreversible and the ovaries will never again work as they once did.

Modern medical advances have come out of the desire to ensure that fertility is preserved for women undergoing chemotherapy. There are several new (and expensive) therapies that can either save a frozen embryo to be implanted after treatment, or preserve ovarian tissue to be re-implanted after treatment.

You may want to consider having your eggs harvested for an IVF procedure with your partner's sperm. Embryos can be frozen and transferred back either into your own uterus (if you haven't had a hysterectomy) or into a surrogate's uterus. In June of 2005, McGill University in Montreal announced the successful birth of a baby boy born as the result of IVF using frozen eggs, and this procedure has also been performed in the US. In this procedure a woman's eggs are removed and flash-frozen before her chemotherapy treatment. The eggs are stored until the woman is ready to become pregnant. At that time, the eggs are thawed and doctors use IVF to achieve fertilization. This technique allows women to maintain fertility even if they aren't currently in a relationship.

Infertility experts in the US have had some recent success in their attempts to preserve fertility in female chemotherapy patients by removing their ovaries before treatment, and re-implanting the ovarian tissue after treatment.

Premature Menopause

Studies have found that the chemotherapy treatment of GTN usually bumps up the average age of menopause. If you've undergone chemo for GTN and have retained your fertility, you may want to factor the possibility of early menopause into your family planning.

I experienced premature menopause. I had a partial hysterectomy, but then had so many doses of chemo it took a toll on my body. I found it really hard to deal with the moodiness and the hot flashes. I'd wake up in the middle of the night, drenched. I had to change pajamas two to four times in a night. And sometimes during the day I'd get a hot flash in the middle of a conversation with someone, and I wouldn't be able to pay attention to what it was they were saying!

Hysterectomy

If you've had a hysterectomy, it means your womb was removed. It also means that you can no longer carry a baby, since the womb that would house the developing fetus is gone. However, it doesn't mean that you can't become a parent. There are many options available for parenting, even if you've lost your fertility. One option is to adopt. Numerous agencies throughout the world help connect people who want to be parents with young children who have been put up for adoption. However, it's important to be patient, since the adoption process is often very long and involved.

You might also consider contracting with a surrogate mother. A surrogate mother carries a fetus while it's developing, and then gives the baby to the contracting parents after she's given birth. The embryo that's implanted in the surrogate can be genetically related to you, if you've had one of your eggs removed for fertilization with your husband's sperm. Other couples have used donated eggs, fertilized with the husband's sperm. Still others have used both donated eggs and donated sperm.

After my hysterectomy, I was very lucky and grateful to be alive, but devastated that I wouldn't be able to have any more children. TJ and I talked and cried about this (we already had names picked out for our next one or two kids). And then we talked about surrogacy as well as adoption and fostering. Surrogacy is a lot more expensive, because you have to pay for the in-vitro fertilization (mixing your husband's sperm and your eggs in a petri dish). In some countries you also have to pay the surrogate mother (who is the woman willing to carry and deliver your child). Adoption is worth considering, given the number of children out there who've been given up, left behind or taken away from unfit parents. Fostering is also great because there are so many kids out there who just need a little guidance, as well as those who are older and can't find a family willing to adopt them. We realized that it didn't matter whether or not I could physically carry and give birth to a child; our opportunities as parents were endless.

CHEMOTHERAPY RESISTANCE

Chemotherapy resistance refers to a situation in which diseased placental cells become unresponsive to chemotherapy treatment. It isn't known exactly why this occurs. You may have heard of patients with other forms of cancer who've developed chemotherapy resistance, which then complicated their treatment. However, one of the striking features of gestational trophoblastic neoplasias is that they respond well to treatment. Even patients who develop chemotherapy resistance can often be successfully treated once they change their regimens (see pages 89–90 for more on treating resistant GTN). While the thought of developing chemotherapy resistance may seem frightening, it's important to understand that between 70 to 100 percent of patients still achieve remission even after developing chemotherapy resistance during their treatment.

Chemo resistance happens when you're on a certain protocol for long periods of time, or if you've been treated with the same drug before (and your body has become used to it). This is what happened in my case, and as a result I was on three different chemo protocols. Sometimes, when there's a minimal amount of diseased placental cells left in your body, the placental cells may "hide" from a particular type of chemo, making it hard for the chemo to reach them and kill them off.

Only one of the women interviewed developed chemotherapy resistance:

> "The first time I was on methotrexate, and my hCG levels went from 3,000 up to 4,000. My doctor called me at work on a Friday at 3 p.m., and told me that my levels [had gone] up, and [that I had to] to come in right away to re-do bloodwork. The next Monday I started on actinomycin-D. [for the] second time. My levels dropped very slowly on actinomycin-D [and] after three months I was given the opportunity once again to get a hysterectomy or go on EMA-CO." (Diagnosed at 41 in 1999; treated in Memphis, TN, then Fort Lauderdale, FL.)

GTN RECURRENCE

Sometimes gestational trophoblastic neoplasia comes back even after a doctor has declared that you're in remission. It's not known why some people experience recurrence, while others do not. Recurrence happens in about 2.5 percent of women with nonmetastatic GTN, 3.7 percent of women with low-risk metastatic GTN and 13 percent of women with high-risk metastatic GTN. Almost all recurrences take place within three years of remission (85 percent recur in the first 18 months). However, sometimes GTN may recur a long time later, even after a normal, full-term pregnancy.

Recurrent gestational trophoblastic neoplasia is usually treated with chemotherapy. The fact that you've had a recurrence places you in the high-risk category, regardless of what risk category you were assigned at the time of your first diagnosis. Recurrent GTN is treated in the same manner as high-risk choriocarcinoma (see pages 87–89 for more information on high-risk treatment).

Here's what the women we spoke with told us about their experience of recurrence:

> "After chemotherapy had been finished for about eight months, my hCG went up quickly. They thought it was a recurrence and I returned to chemotherapy. When we were almost finished with the therapies my doctor discovered that it may have been caused by something he called "the hormonal surge." He changed the birth control pill he had me on, and my hCG went below 1. We did finish the chemotherapies because I only had two more to go, and we knew we would hate ourselves if he was wrong." (Diagnosed at 31 in 1994; treated in Cleveland, OH.)

> "Yes. First time of course, and I'll never forget the exact moment. I went in for a check-up at the oncologist's, and he asked why I hadn't gotten weekly bloodwork. I told him I had five in a row that were less than 2, and no one told me to continue weekly. Three days later I got a call to come back in and re-test. I immediately drove 30 miles to the doctor's in a terrible panic. On January 5th my hCG was less than 2; on January 29th it was 86. So I don't know when it came back, [but] I assume [it was] about four to five weeks post chemo (I finished chemo on December 12th 2000). The second time [was] exactly three and a half weeks post chemo—recurrence again. Again my hCG was 86 (whereas

10 days earlier [it had been] less than 2). My feelings the first time were: 'Oh, they just didn't get it all.' The second time, I knew the battle was over. I felt defeat, and extreme anxiety. I was in the hospital having a hysterectomy within two weeks of that reading. I was so sad and worn out and, looking back, suffered immense grief, although I didn't let myself grieve fully then. I wish I'd been offered counseling. I kept a lot bottled up inside." (Diagnosed at 41 in 1999; treated in Memphis, TN, then Fort Lauderdale, FL.)

LONG-TERM COMPLICATIONS OF TREATMENT

Some of the chemotherapy drugs used in the treatment of GTN can put you at increased risk of developing some forms of cancer later on in life (leukemia, colon cancer and breast cancer). Cancers that occur after chemotherapy treatment are called "secondary cancers." Secondary tumors are known to occur with the use of etoposide, actinomycin-D and cyclophosphamide.

That said, chemotherapy is still one of the best methods of treatment we have available right now. So the small risk of developing a secondary cancer must be balanced against chemotherapy's ability to achieve remission. If you've been treated with chemotherapy, it's important to remain vigilant about screening for these other forms of cancer. Get into the habit of performing regular breast self-examinations, and let your family doctor know about any treatments you've had in the past. He or she should be aware that screening for these secondary forms of cancer is crucial.

DEATH

When people are first told that they have cancer, thoughts of death often come to mind. Many GTN patients experience these fears, even when they have a mild non-cancerous form of the disease. GTN patients may fear that their disease will progress to become choriocarcinoma. For the majority of patients with GTN and choriocarcinoma, these fears are unfounded. The cure rates for GTN and choriocarcinoma are high; between 75 and 100 percent of GTN and chorio patients can expect a full recovery. However, if you're one of the 25 percent who have complications associated with therapy, these statistics will be of little comfort.

I constantly thought about death. I really didn't want to die. I thought about how my family would cope with it, and what would happen if I did die. I felt I had to talk to TJ about things like how I'd rather be cremated, and how I'd rather no funeral service. I had to talk about him remarrying. I talked about all of this so much TJ started to get mad at me for being such a downer. I can see his point of view though, wanting to be optimistic about everything, or just not wanting to talk about the bad stuff (because if we did, then it was bound to happen).

There were days I felt I'd rather die than feel the way I did. I'm really glad I fought as hard as I did—I guess I had no choice. But I was mentally and physically exhausted, and would have been prepared if I were to just pass away. It took me a long time to actually admit this, and it makes me cry just thinking about it now. I think I was more at peace with my chances—the idea that I was in a lower percentile (in terms of survival) than all of my family and friends. I'd wanted all or nothing, basically to feel really good, or be gone.

After a year of chemo, I think anyone would be ready to give up. Don't. Those who've been through this know how tough it is. Some of the women we interviewed at the Yahoo support group have been in treatment for three months; others for 6 years. We're all still here.

You might want to consider some of the mechanics of actually dealing with death. These all need to be addressed well in advance because it's impossible to do so on the deathbed.

- You may want to write letters or prepare some videos for your children to have later. Some hospitals include services to help you prepare these documents, or you can simply prepare them on your own.
- Be sure that you have an up-to-date will that outlines how you'd like your estate to be distributed. You can consult with a lawyer to help you prepare your will, or there may be do-it-yourself "will kits" available in your area.
- In some cases (for example, if you are divorced or a single mother) you may want to clarify who will have custody of your children in the event of your death.

Talking to Children About Death and Saying Goodbye

Questions about Death

Questions about death are often the most difficult to address. Unfortunately, whatever preparing you do may not help you feel ready to answer the actual questions when they arise. Furthermore, even if you give the "right" answer, you may feel like you should have said more. Don't be too hard on yourself. Remember that thinking about death is difficult not only for a child, but also for you. If you feel that you really can't talk about death with your child, then it may be helpful to enlist the help of a counselor who specializes in talking to kids about death in the family.

At the time of this writing, Meredith worked at the Hospital for Sick Children in Toronto. She attended several seminars on talking to children about death, and heard all the tips for maintaining open communication. Yet when Tara's son, Tragean, asked her about death she found answering very difficult. Tragean approached her and said: "Meredith, I heard that sometimes people die in their sleep. My mom sleeps all the time and it makes me worried." Meredith wanted to open the conversation to the topic of death. She knew she should validate Tragean's concerns by saying something like: "Well, it's natural to be worried; sometimes people do die in their sleep. But the kind of cancer that your mom has is one that people usually recover from..." When faced with the question in real life, however, all she could come up with was a forceful: "Your mom won't die. When you mom sleeps, it doesn't mean she's going to die. It just means she needs to rest so she can get better." Meredith felt that her answer was inadequate, yet she couldn't bring herself to admit (even to herself) that death was a possibility.

Parents often worry that, in addressing their kids' questions about death, they'll convey their own uncertainty, or their hopelessness about the future. It may help to acknowledge that your child's fear is normal, and that sometimes cancer can kill people (it's best not to lie about this). But you can also be clear about the fact that you intend to take good care of yourself (or if the father is talking to them, that he intends to take good care of mommy), and that you're pursuing the best available treatments and will probably recover. Acknowledge how difficult it is to deal with uncertainty. You might say something like: "Uncertainty means hoping for the best and having a back-up plan for the worst. Do you have any worries or questions about what will happen to you if I died?" Exploring the back-up plan together may help the child feel more secure (e.g., you might talk about who'll take care of them in the event of your death, so that they won't worry they'll be left alone). You can also use this opportunity to stress that the well parent will continue to love and care for them.

When I first found out that I had chorio, I was really scared to tell Tragean. I had to wait for the perfect time so I could explain it and deal with his reactions without crying myself. I had to be strong. Just a couple of days before I told him, we were watching a TV show. One of the kids on this show had leukemia when she was younger, and had been moody that week because her yearly check-up was approaching. Tragean asked what leukemia was and I told him that it was a type of cancer. His eyes got wide, and he whispered: "You can die from that." My reply was: "Yes, you can but that girl has beaten it and is all better." So, when the time came to tell Tragean, I brought up the day we all went to the doctor, the day I came out of the doctor's office crying. I told him that I'd been crying because I'd just been told I had cancer. I told him that the doctors were trying their hardest to make me better, but that the medication I'd be on would make me a lot more sick before it would make me better. He had the same stupid grin on his face as I did when I was first told about my diagnosis. He asked me if I was going to die. This was a really tough question, and he asked it of me a lot when I was going through treatments. I always replied: "If I have my way, I'm not going to die." Not only did that make him feel better, it made me feel better too.

Saying Goodbye

If something goes wrong in your treatment you may have to let your children know. This can be incredibly difficult. What you want your children to know and remember must be stated explicitly and repeatedly until you're satisfied that they've absorbed it. You might want to let them know that you love them, that you don't want to leave, that it isn't their fault, and that you really want them to be happy. If your children know that they're loved, then you may not actually have to say goodbye.

If it's possible for your children to say their last "I love yous" in person, it may help to make the death more real. If it isn't possible for them to say "I love you" before death, this goodbye can occur at the funeral, or privately at the funeral home.

At the bedside the children should be invited to express their final thoughts to the parent. If the dying parent is in a coma, an adult may want to tell the children something like: "We don't know what people in a coma can hear, but we believe they can feel the presence of other family members." This may be a good time for the family to remember incidents that capture the spirit of the dying parent. Surprisingly, the stories that unfold are often humorous or bittersweet.

Sometimes children fear that they'll forget the dying parent, so it's important to reassure them that there will be people around to remind them of how the dying parent looked, or how she would have responded to a given situation.

A trusted adult might also let your children know that it will take a long while for the empty spot in their hearts to feel better, but that they may find the dead parent is still a presence for them in hard times. Children may react surprisingly well, since they're already used to the sadness of a long-term illness. Remind the children how strong they've been in coping with the illness until now, and try to convey the confidence you feel about their ability to go forward. Remind them that the dead parent would want them to stay engaged, and to stay in the world of the living. It's important to help children feel that they're not being disloyal to the dead parent if and when they finally have a moment during which they're able to forget their grief.

Grieving parents can assist their children by asking about the specifics of school, friends, sports and other activities. Attention to these details delivers the message that the surviving parent values normality, and that the children are supported in their efforts to reinvest in their lives. If the grieving parent is having a hard time adjusting himself, then it may be a good idea to enlist the help of friends, family, or even a professional counselor.

CHAPTER 9

RECOVERY AND BEYOND

DELAYED REACTIONS TO THE DIAGNOSIS OF GTN

Many women who are currently going through diagnosis and treatment for gestational trophoblastic neoplasia and choriocarcinoma don't have the time or energy to deal with their feelings about being sick. All their energy is focused on getting better. Once treatments have finished and they're in remission, these women find themselves overwhelmed with emotion. Patients often report that they go through a period of depression *after* treatments finish. At this point they want to return to life as usual, yet they're faced with continuing uncertainty, and the fear of recurrence. Even patients who've achieved remission or cure have a higher prevalence of anxiety and depression than what's considered normal in the general population. Furthermore, moving from treatment to remission is another adjustment that dramatically affects personal relationships.

Patients report that the excitement of finishing treatment is often intermingled with exhaustion and fear. For these patients a sense of safety and security is difficult to recapture. They feel restless or irritable, easily fatigued, and they worry excessively and experience sleep disturbances and/or panic attacks. They may be embarrassed about their ongoing depression and anxiety, and they may put pressure on themselves to "get over it." They may feel guilty about the time it's taking them to return to normal. These experiences are so common and so ultimately significant that some authors now suggest the post-cancer experience is similar to the post-traumatic stress experienced by victims of rape or war. It's clear that recovery from GTN doesn't stop at remission or cure. However, with time, you should begin to feel better. If you find you're continually afraid, consider seeing a counselor or psychotherapist who can help you work through these difficult emotions.

As I write this, I consider the fact that it's been almost four months since my last treatment, and that there's an abundance of emotion swirling around in this house! I found that when I was trying to get better, I was so caught up in the moment (and in everything I wanted to learn and remember) that my real life was put on hold. After my treatment ended, I didn't know which way was up. I was lost without the hustle and bustle of going in and out of the cancer center and the hospital. And I had no idea where to start my life again. I wanted to know that if I *did* start there'd be no recurrence. But there's just no guarantee. I had to get back to caring for my family, regaining my strength, and becoming my old self once again. TJ and I had to rekindle our relationship too, since it was basically put on hold for a good part of my chemo.

Here's an entry from my journal, which was written one month before I finished my last treatment. At the time, I was trying to put my life back on track, and yet I didn't know when I'd be in remission, or when I'd finish treatment:

"I'm feeling lost, overwhelmed, and scared. I'm feeling like I don't know what I'm feeling. Lost in limbo. Lost somewhere: in the past, in the future. Trying to find my path: any path, the right path. I want to make everything better. I want to get over what happened. Get on with my life. But what if? So many what ifs. What if there were no what ifs? Could I get on with my life then? Or would I still feel this way?"

This book made sure that I relived many of the moments when I was sick. Which has been great, since only now am I able to physically and mentally deal with them. I now realize what I've actually been through, and it amazes me to see how well I handled everything that I had to face. Now I understand why everyone says that I'm a very strong person. I doubted that statement for a very long time. Now I think of it and smile.

PREGNANCY AFTER GTN TREATMENT

If your treatment did not involve a hysterectomy, you may be wondering about your chances of having a normal pregnancy after treatment. The good news is that patients with gestational trophoblastic neoplasia can usually achieve complete remission while retaining their fertility, even when there has been widespread metastasis. One study found that 68.6 percent of patients with complete moles and 74.1 percent of patients with partial moles were able to have a normal pregnancy after treatment for GTN. After one molar pregnancy, your risk of repeating the experience is only 1 percent (which is somewhat higher than that of the general population, where risk is about 1 in 1,000). However, if you've had two molar pregnancies, then you actually have a 23 percent chance of experiencing a third. Patients who've undergone chemotherapy for persistent gestational trophoblastic tumors had normal pregnancies following treatment 68.6 percent of the time.

Since the risk of having a subsequent molar pregnancy is somewhat higher if you've already had one, it's important to let your obstetrician know about previous GTN treatment. You should have an ultrasound in the first trimester to confirm that normal development is taking place. Before you give birth you should let the doctor who is delivering know about your previous experience with GTN and ask him or her to thoroughly examine the placenta and products of conception for any possible pathology. Six weeks after you've given birth you should have your hCG levels checked to rule out recurrent GTN or choriocarcinoma.

You should also avoid becoming pregnant for one year after you finish treatment for GTN. During this period your doctor will want to monitor your hCG levels to ensure that you're free of disease. A pregnancy makes it difficult to monitor hCG levels, since this hormone increases during gestation. If you do get pregnant while your hCG levels are still being monitored, you can continue your pregnancy. Most patients (75.9 percent) who became pregnant before their follow-up is complete have normal pregnancies and deliveries. A few (10.3 percent) have normal pregnancies with preterm deliveries.

Here's one woman's story about pregnancy after chorio treatment:

> "I had a boy three years after treatment, and a girl five years after. They're three and one now. They were normal pregnancies apart from the initial worry." (Diagnosed at 30 in 1997; treated in Sheffield, UK.)

Some patients worry about their chances of a repeat experience with GTN; however, studies have shown that in the majority of cases women have been able to have a normal pregnancy after being treated for GTN. There are emotional worries associated with a pregnancy after GTN (or any other form of pregnancy loss). Both women and their husbands have reported greater feelings of anxiety about a pregnancy that follows GTN. Women who miscarried have reported that they were slower to grow attached to the second pregnancy because they were afraid that something would go wrong again. Every symptom or event during the pregnancy made them anxious.

Some women become extra-vigilant in their self-care during the subsequent pregnancy; they try to do everything they can to ensure a better outcome this time. Some women feel responsible for the health of their fetus, and worry that if they experience GTN again, they'll somehow be at fault. Some women express fears about not being able to cope if they lose another baby due to GTN. And many women feel that they didn't receive enough support from others concerning their fears about their new pregnancy. Instead, people tended to dismiss it, and quote statistics about how unlikely it was for GTN to recur. Rather than feeling reassured, women experienced this as dismissive of *their* experience.

However, feelings about a new pregnancy are not all negative. Many women talk about how hopeful they feel that things will work out this time (though their optimism is somewhat guarded, as they constantly fear bad news).

Prospective fathers' feelings about a pregnancy following GTN have not been well studied. Prospective fathers' experiences of pregnancy after miscarriage are often overlooked, as researchers tend to focus on the experience of the prospective mother. However, fathers, too, have mixed feelings about a pregnancy that occurs after treatment for GTN. When the mothers' and fathers' reactions are compared, studies have found that the fathers tend to be more hopeful than the mothers, and less influenced by the previous loss of pregnancy once a new pregnancy has occurred.

Prospective fathers might deny their own emotional reactions in an attempt to protect and support their wives. Fathers seem to have less of a desire for support during a pregnancy following GTN than do their wives. However, fathers do express emotions about the new pregnancy, which they attribute to the previous loss. These emotions include an increased concern related to the outcome of the new pregnancy, a heightened sense of risk since the loss, a realization that something could go wrong with the new pregnancy, and a need for increased vigilance in the new pregnancy. See the resource list at the back of this book for websites that discuss miscarriage.

LIFE AS A SURVIVOR

Life as a survivor of a life-threatening disease can be very different. Many survivors report a shift in their priorities. They no longer "sweat the small stuff." Many report that they feel brave and are more likely to "just do it." Life is too short to put things off. Survivors also often report that they feel more confident when confronted with difficult situations. They know that

able to handle tough times in the past, and that they'll be able
gain.

ng this now, I consider that it's been almost two years since I was
first diagnosed, and I'm still going for bloodwork every two weeks. My hCG
count has been at less then 2 for the past two months, and I'm starting to
get used to the idea that this whole ordeal may be over. I still get butterflies
before hearing the results of my bloodwork, just hoping that I don't have to
go through it all again. But I'm working a full- and a part-time job right now,
as well as raising my kids and hubby!

I found that finishing my last treatment and trying to get my life back to
normal was really hard emotionally. I had to take a leap (and it was a big one)
to get out there—to get a job and try to live normally without worrying about
whether or not the cancer would recur. Now I'm able to enjoy an evening
out with my friends. I'm able to laugh, dance and chitchat, take my family
to the beach, swim and play Frisbee. I'm also enjoying the taste of food again
(I knew my husband could cook!), though for a long while it seemed like
nothing I ate was enjoyable.

Here is what some of the women we interviewed had to say about life
as a survivor:

> "I'm definitely more spiritual, and I eliminate the things in my
> life that are unimportant. I try to live life to the fullest and don't
> associate with people who aren't positive, or those who bring me
> down. I'm less afraid to take chances." (Diagnosed at 33 in 2000;
> treated in Toronto, Canada.)

> "[Life as a survivor is] wonderful! I do appreciate things more, like
> beauty in nature, time with friends and family, continued good
> health. I also have less patience for complainers and mean people.
> My husband says I'm more vocal about my feelings, and more as-
> sertive in dealing with people. I could go on and on. The biggest
> change physically has been the toll on my body. I feel as though I
> aged five years in two—but I guess "older and wiser" applies now!"
> (Diagnosed at 41 in 1999; treated in Memphis, TN, then Fort
> Lauderdale, FL.)

> "My husband and I have a better marriage now than we ever had
> before. I believe the cancer had a lot to do with this." (Diagnosed
> at 31 in 1994; treated in Cleveland, OH.)

Parting Thoughts

Tara

When I first moved back to Saskatoon, I was still undergoing treatment and didn't know how much longer it would continue. A few months later, a friend of ours suggested we take a trip to Shuswap Lake in British Columbia, to go houseboating. TJ and I were all for it, and jumped at the chance to go. We organized everything, and actually rounded up a group of 22 people (of which Meredith was a part!). I was pumped about this trip, and promised myself that I'd be finished treatment by the time we had to leave (the middle of June).

It was great to have something to look forward to. And I kept my promise: I finished my last treatment April 5th 2003. It was also great to see Meredith again; we had a blast! I felt like my old self. Even my hair had started to grow back (I looked like a little boy, but who cares; I had hair!). I definitely needed the vacation, and was better able to relax and get into the swing of things when I got back home. It was so much fun we decided to go again the following year.

Meredith

I was really excited to see Tara again. After she moved back to Saskatchewan, we saw each other very rarely. I knew at the time of her move that I'd miss her whole family very much. They'd become such a big part of my life. But I wasn't prepared for the joy I felt when I arrived at the lake, and saw Tara on the dock. She looked so healthy!

We climbed a mountain together on that trip. It was an amazing experience to be up there, to look out over a waterfall with my best friend. She couldn't even move about her apartment without taking breaks the last time I saw her. Now here she was: strong and beautiful and climbing the Rockies. TJ and I were the ones struggling to keep up.

RESOURCE LIST

Support Groups

A Choriocarcinoma Support Group at Yahoo (formerly choriocarcinoma at Yahoo Clubs): Information and support.
http://groups.yahoo.com/group/AChoriocarcinomaSupportGroup/

MyMolarPregnancy.com: Personal stories, information, and support.
www.mymolarpregnancy.com

Eyes on the Prize: Information and emotional support from the survivors' perspective.
www.eyesontheprize.org

Support Groups for Dealing with Miscarriage

SilentGrief.com: An online support group. The site also contains information for fathers who are going through miscarriage in the "articles" section.
www.silentgrief.com/

Angel Babies Forever Loved: This website features a chatroom on Monday evenings from 9-11 p.m. EST.
www.angels4ever.com/

Miscarriage Support Auckland Inc: This site includes information on men and women's reactions to miscarriage, and the differences between them.
www.miscarriagesupport.org.nz/together.html

Useful Websites Related to Choriocarcinoma and GTN

University of New Mexico Health Sciences Center & School of Medicine: Department of OB/GYN Women's Health Research: This website provides a list of doctors and a lot of information about hCG testing.
www.hcglab.com

Charing Cross Site on Hydatidiform Mole & Choriocarcinoma: Don't be afraid to check out the information for medics as well as the information for patients.
www.hmole-chorio.org.uk/

B.C. Cancer Agency Drug Manual: This site has a complete listing of drugs used to treat cancers of all types. You can look up the drugs you are prescribed here.
www.bccancer.bc.ca/HPI/DrugDatabase/DrugIndexALPt/default.htm

Dr. William Rich's GTD and Gynecological Cancer site:
www.gyncancer.com

International Society for the Study of Trophoblastic Diseases (ISSTD): This site contains a lot of information, including an online book.
www.isstd.org/

Women's Cancer Network:
www.wcn.org

National Cancer Institute:
www.cancer.gov

Useful Web Resources for Complementary and Alternative Therapy Research

Quackwatch: The site is designed to help you make informed intelligent decisions about the use of CAMs.
www.quackwatch.org/

BC Cancer Agency: Information for patients and their families, relating to alternative and complementary therapies.
www.bccancer.bc.ca/PPI/UnconventionalTherapies/default.htm

The Canadian Health Network (CHN): This site provides reliable information on CAMs and also contains a frequently asked questions page.
www.canadianhealthcarenetwork.ca

GLOSSARY

Adjuvant Chemotherapy: The use of chemotherapy as an adjuvant therapy (see below).

Adjuvant Therapy: A treatment method used in addition to the primary therapy to improve the chances of curing cancer.

Alopecia: The loss of hair from the body and/or scalp.

Anemia: A medical term that means low red blood cell count. Symptoms of anemia are fatigue and shortness of breath.

Angiogenesis: The development of new capillary blood vessels.

Anorexia: The loss of appetite for food.

Antiangiogenic: Therapies that are aimed at stopping the growth of new blood vessels so that the cancer will "starve" and die.

Anti-emetic: A medicine used to relieve nausea and/or vomiting.

Apoptosis: Purposeful cell death, sometimes called cell suicide. The cell dies to prevent the spread of genetic "mistakes."

Autonomy: The patient's right to make her own decisions about healthcare treatments.

Benign: A tumor that is localized, has not spread and for which treatment is expected to produce a cure; the opposite of malignant.

Biopsy: A piece of body tissue removed from a patient for further study.

Blastocyst: The name of the stage of the developing baby at about day five, when the developing baby has reached the uterus.

Blood Tests: A test in which blood is drawn and examined under a microscope and/or by reacting it with chemicals to determine whether different substances are present in the blood.

Blood Vessels: Any tube in the body that carries blood. Arteries, arterioles, capillaries, veins and veuels are all different types of blood vessels.

Bone Marrow: The soft, spongy tissue in bone cavities. Bone marrow is where red blood cells, white blood cells and platelets develop.

Cancer: The uncontrolled, abnormal growth of cells that can invade and destroy healthy body tissues and organs. Most cancers can also spread to other parts of the body.

Carcinogenesis: The process by which normal cells become cancerous.

CAT Scan: See "Computed Tomography."

CBC: Complete blood count.

Chemotherapy: Means "drug treatment" but the term usually refers to the treatment of cancer with drugs. Commonly called "chemo." This is a systemic treatment because the drugs enter the bloodstream and travel through the body to kill cancer cells found in any organ.

Chorioadenoma Destruens: Another name for invasive mole (see "Hydatidiform Mole").

Choriocarcinogenesis: The development of choriocarcinoma from healthy placental cells.

Choriocarcinoma (or Gestational Choriocarcinoma): From "chorion," which is one of the protective layers around the embryo and "carcinoma," which indicates a type of cancer that forms in the lining (or epithelium) of body organs (rather than deep in organ tissues). Commonly called "chorio." A cancer that develops from fetal placental tissues, choriocarcinoma spreads rapidly, but it is usually quite responsive to chemotherapy.

Chorion: The membrane that surrounds and protects the embryo.

Chromosomes: Chromosomes are self-replicating genetic structures, which contain the DNA.

Combination Chemotherapy: Treatment that consists of several anticancer drugs given at the same time.

Computed Tomography (CT Scan or CAT Scan): A special X-ray procedure that uses a computer to assimilate multiple X-ray images into a two dimensional cross-section. These tests can detect more soft tissue structures than a single X-ray can by itself.

Congenital Conditions: A condition is congenital when it is present at birth. Congenital conditions are not necessarily genetic.

Contraindication: A reason not to use a particular drug or treatment.

CT Scan: See "Computed Tomography."

Cyst: A sac filled with fluid; may be normal or abnormal.

Cytotrophoblast: One of the three types of trophoblast (placental) cells.

Delirium: Disturbances of attention, thinking, perception, judgment, emotion and memory. Delirium can also be accompanied by disorientation (this side effect has been referred to by patients as "chemo brain").

Diagnosis: The determination of the nature or cause of the symptoms, signs or disease about which the patient complains.

Dilation and Curettage (D & C): An operation that stretches the cervix (the opening of the uterus). The walls of the uterus are then scraped to remove endometrial material.

Discharge: A fluid that is released from the body.

DNA: Short for deoxyribonucleic acid; refers to the molecule that encodes the genetic material that is found in the nucleus of every human cell. The DNA contains instructions for controlling the development, structure and function of all cells.

Dysfunction: Abnormal function; not working properly.

Dysmenorrhea: Painful menstruation; cramps.

Dyspareunia: Pain during sexual intercourse.

E-cadherin: A cell adhesion molecule. It is believed that damage to this molecule might lead to a tumor's ability to spread (metastasize).

Eclampsia: A more severe form of preeclampsia. See "Preeclampsia."

Ectopic pregnancy: The development of the fetus in the fallopian tube, or other abnormal location, instead of in the uterus.

Embryo: The stage in the development of a baby during which the cells are dividing most rapidly. From about two weeks until the end of the seventh or eighth week.

Endometrium: The inner lining of the uterus where the initial attachment of the embryo occurs; a portion of this lining is shed each month with menstruation.

Enzymes: Allow chemical reactions to begin. Enzymes "jump start" the reaction.

Erythema: A reddening of the skin that is caused by clogged capillaries.

Esophagus: The part of the digestive system that connects the mouth to the stomach.

Estrogen (Oestrogen): Female hormone produced by the ovarian follicles.

Familial Conditions: Conditions that occur in several members of a family are called familial. Often assumed to be genetic, but this is not always the case.

Fertilization: The union of the male gamete (sperm) with the female gamete (egg).

Fetus: The developing baby during the stage when it begins to take on a recognizable form, which is from about the end of the seventh or eight week until it is born.

Fever: A rise in body temperature of above 38ºC or 100.4ºF, though this number may vary somewhat from person to person. Often in response to an infection.

Gamete (Germ Cell): Reproductive cell; the sperm in men, the egg in women.

Gastrointestinal (GI): The digestive system, including the stomach and intestines.

Gene: The unit of heredity, composed of DNA; the building block of chromosomes.

Genetic: A general term that is used to discuss conditions that arise because of genes or chromosomes.

Genotype: The genetic make-up of an organism, as distinct from the expressed features (what the organism looks like and how it behaves, a.k.a. phenotype).

Gestation Sac: The fluid-filled sac in which the fetus develops, visible by an ultrasound exam. Sometimes called the amniotic sac.

Gestation: Pregnancy.

Gestational Trophoblastic Disease (GTD): The old name for gestational trophoblastic neoplasia (GTN). Please see "Gestational Trophoblastic Neoplasia (GTN)."

Gestational Trophoblastic Neoplasia (GTN): A disease associated with pregnancy. GTN is actually a group of several diseases: hydatidiform mole, invasive mole, persistent Gestational Trophoblastic Neoplasia, choriocarcinoma and placental-site trophoblastic tumor. All these diseases involve abnormally growing cells inside a woman's uterus in which the abnormal growth develops from cells associated with an embryo, rather than from the cells of the uterus itself.

Gland: An organ that produces and secretes essential body fluids or substances, such as hormones.

Gonads: Organs that produce the sex cells and sex hormones; testicles in men and ovaries in women.

Gynecological Oncologist (Gyn-Onc): A doctor who specializes in cancers of the female reproductive system (uterus, ovaries, cervix and vagina).

hCG: Please see "Human Chorionic Gonadotropin."

Hormone: A substance, produced by an endocrine gland, which travels through the bloodstream to a specific organ, where it exerts its effect.

Human Chorionic Gonadotropin (hCG): A hormone associated with pregnancy (the hormone that is detected by home pregnancy tests). hCG helps regulate the proper balance of ovarian hormone production during pregnancy. Produced by the placental cells.

Human Placental Lactogen (hPL): This hormone is involved in preparing breast tissue for lactation, or milk production. Produced by the placental cells. This hormone can sometimes be a marker for a placental site trophoblastic tumor.

Hydatidiform Mole, Complete: A mole that contains no fetal tissue. May develop into a cancerous form of GTN.

Hydatidiform Mole, Invasive: A hydatidiform mole that penetrates the myometrium (the muscular wall of the uterus). If the tumor grows through the full thickness of the myometrium it may result in a hole in the uterus that may lead to heavy bleeding.

Hydatidiform Mole, Partial: A mole that contains some tissue from an abnormal fetus with multiple malformations. The fetus usually spontaneously aborts. Partial moles rarely develop into cancerous forms of GTN.

Hydatidiform Mole: From "hyd," which means water. This refers to the fact that hydatidiform moles are shaped like water droplets or grapes.

Hyperplastic: Tissue that grows excessively.

Hyperthyroidism: An over-active thyroid gland, which is producing an excess of thyroid hormone. This syndrome is characterized by enlarged thyroid gland (in the neck), warm skin tremors and feelings of restlessness.

Hypoxia: The reduction of the oxygen supply to tissues below the normal levels necessary for functioning, despite the presence of an adequate blood supply.

Hysterectomy: The surgical removal of the uterus.

Hysterosalpingogram (HSG): An X-ray examination in which a dye is injected into the uterus to illustrate the inner contour of the uterus and degree of openness of the uterine tubes.

Hysteroscope: A telescopic device, which enables examination of the uterine cavity.

Immune System: The body's defense against any injury or invasion by a foreign substance or organism.

Immunoglobulins: A class of proteins that fight infection; antibodies.

Implantation: Attachment of the fertilized egg to the uterine lining, usually occurring five to seven days after ovulation.

Infection: The invasion and multiplication of microorganisms (such as bacteria) in body tissues.

Inflammation: A response to some type of injury such as infection, characterized by increased blood flow, heat, redness, swelling, and pain.

Intermediate Trophoblast: One of the three types of trophoblast (placental) cells. Involved in the production of human placental lactogen (hPL).

Karyotype: A chromosome analysis.

Labia (Majora and Minora): Two folds of tissue ("lips") that surround the vaginal opening.

Laparoscope: A thin instrument with a telescopic lens, which a surgeon inserts through the body wall and uses to view internal organs and abdominal cavity.

Leukorrhea: Whitish, mucousy vaginal discharge, common during pregnancy.

Luteomas: A benign tumor on the ovaries.

Malignant: A tumor that has become invasive and has the potential to have metastases (spread). These types of tumors are considered cancerous. The opposite of benign.

Mesoderm: The embryonic tissue layer that gives rise to muscle, organs, most of the internal skeleton and connective tissue.

Miscarriage: The spontaneous loss of a pregnancy.

Mitosis: The process by which the body grows and replaces damaged body tissues. This term is often used interchangeably with cell division.

Molar Pregnancy: A pregnancy that has no embryo, but rather a mole, or cluster of grape-like cells.

Mole: Please see "Hydatidiform Mole."

Morula: The name of the developing baby immediately after conception. This stage lasts about four days until the Blastocyst stage.

Motility: Motion.

Mucus: Secretion from a gland that can be watery, gel-like, stretchy, sticky or dry.

Multifactorial (or Complex) Genetic Diseases: In these diseases there is an inherited contribution, but this only becomes relevant in combination with lifestyle and other environmental causes.

Myometrium: The muscular wall of the uterus. These muscles are used during the birthing process to expel the fetus out of the womb and into the world.

Neoadjuvant Chemotherapy: A form of adjuvant chemotherapy that is given before the primary form of treatment.

Neoplasia (Neoplasm): Means "new growth"; another word used to refer to cancer. It has the same meaning as tumor, and likewise can be benign or malignant.

Nongestational Choriocarcinoma: In extremely rare instances choriocarcinoma can develop in other parts of the body unrelated to pregnancy. In these cases choriocarcinoma is usually mixed with other types of cancer. It can be found in the ovaries, testicles, chest or abdomen. (We do not discuss nongestational choriocarcinoma in this book.)

Nonmetastatic: Meaning, the cancer has not spread to organs other than the one in which it originated (it is localized).

Obstetrician-Gynecologist (OBGYN): A physician who specializes in the treatment of female disorders and pregnancy

Oestrogen (Estrogen): Female hormone produced by the ovarian follicles.

Oligomenorrhea: Infrequent and irregular menstrual cycles

Oncogenes: These are genes that play a role in the growth of cells. Their function is to repair body tissues, but when something goes wrong they may cause the cell to grow out of control. When they are signaling growth in the proper way these genes are called proto-oncogenes.

Oncologist: A doctor who specializes in understanding and treating cancer.

Oncology: The study of cancer and the ways to treat cancer.

Organ: A part or structure of an organism that is essential to its survival.

Ovaries: The structures in which eggs (ova) are developed and released during ovulation. Also produce estrogen and progesterone.

Ovulation: The release of an egg from the ovary

Ovum (Ova; Egg): Mature egg.

Oxytocin: A neuropeptide (brain chemical) produced in the brain; stimulates uterine contractions when the mother is giving birth; and causes milk ejection during lactation.

Palliative Care (Palliation): Treatment whose aim is to relieve the symptoms of disease when cancer cannot be cured.

Paralysis: Loss or impairment of motor function, inability to move.

Pathologist: A doctor who examines cells to determine if disease is present.

Peptides: The smaller bits that make up proteins.

Phenotype: The way that a living entity looks or behaves, the result of the interaction between the genes and the environment.

Placenta: The organ that protects and nourishes the growing fetus.

Placental Lactogen: A hormone produced by the placenta that promotes fetal growth.

Placental-Site Trophoblastic Tumor (PSTT): A rare form of GTN that develops at the site where the placenta attaches to the uterus. Most PSTTs do not spread to other sites in the body, though sometimes the tumor will penetrate the muscle layer of the uterus and cause a perforation. PSTTs are not sensitive to chemotherapy drugs, thus treated by complete surgical removal of the uterus.

Polyspermy: Abnormal condition wherein the egg is fertilized by more than one sperm; embryo usually aborts spontaneously due to abnormal chromosomes.

Preeclampsia: A medical condition associated with pregnancy that is characterized by high blood pressure, exaggerated reflexes and excessive blood protein in the urine. When this condition leads to seizures, convulsions or coma the condition is called eclampsia.

Prognosis: A medical prediction of the outcome of an attack, infection or disease; the prospect of recovery.

Prolactin: Pituitary hormone that stimulates milk production

Pronucleus: Specialized nucleus of the egg or sperm.

Proteins: Organic compounds that make up the body tissues.

PSTT: Please see "Placental-Site Trophoblastic Tumor."

Recurrent Cancer: Meaning, the cancer has come back following treatment.

Remission: When the cancer stops spreading and the patient is considered cured.

Salpingectomy: Surgical removal of the fallopian tubes.

Seizure: A sudden attack or convulsion. Characterized by: muscle twitches, staring, tongue biting, urination, loss of consciousness and total body shaking.

Senescence: The normal process that causes a cell to age and eventually to stop replicating and die. Cancer cells lose this process and they keep replicating.

Signs: An indication that something is wrong with the body. Signs are observable by a physician.

Somatic or Acquired Mutations: Bodily cells that are not involved in reproduction (all of the cells other than the sperm or egg cells). These mutations are not passed on to children because they do not affect the sperm and egg cells. For a cell to become cancerous, it usually must acquire more than one somatic mutation.

Symptom: An indication that something is wrong with the body. Symptoms are felt or noticed by the patient, but are not easily observed by anyone else.

Synctiotrophoblast: One of the three types of trophoblastic cells, this produces hCG and helps to produce hPL.

Telomeres: DNA replication cannot start at the very ends of the sequence. In order to avoid losing essential information, the ends of DNA strands contain "nonsense" repeats (telomeres) that do not convey any information. When there is no longer a sufficient length of repeats for complete replication, the cell enters senescence and dies. Cancer cells are able to repair their telomeres so they do not shorten.

Term Pregnancy: A pregnancy that results in a baby.

Trimester: The stages of pregnancy are divided into three parts, with each lasting three months. These parts are called trimesters.

Trophoblast: From "tropho," which means nutrition and "blast," which means bud or early developmental cell. This is the layer of cells that surround the tiny embryo, and in time the trophoblast layer will develop into the placenta. There are three types of trophoblast cells: syncytotiotrophoblast, cytotrophoblast and intermediate trophoblast.

Tumor: An abnormal growth of tissue that can be benign or malignant (cancerous).

Ultrasound (US): Use of high frequency sound waves that can be enlisted painlessly, safely, and without radiation to create an image of internal body parts.

Urination: Going "pee."

Uterus: The hollow, muscular organ in women in which a developing baby is protected and nourished. The uterus opens into the vagina and is protected by a muscular ring called the cervix.

Vagina: The female organ of sexual intercourse; the birth canal.

Vaginal Atrophy: A condition that causes the lining of the vagina to become dry and lose its elasticity.

Vaginal Discharge: A normal white or yellowish fluid (leukorrhea) from the cervical canal or vagina.

Vaginismus: A painful spasmodic contraction of the vagina, which often renders intercourse impossible.

Vaginitis: Inflammation of the vagina.

Villi: Tiny, finger-like projections produced by the trophoblast (placenta) that attach to the lining of the uterus.

Vulva: The visible external parts of the female genitals including the labia and mons pubis, clitoris and opening to the vagina.

X-rays: A type of radiation that can be used at low levels to diagnose disease. In their high-energy form X-rays are used to treat cancer.

Yolk Sac: A membrane that surrounds the developing fetus in the womb.

Zona Pellucida: The protective layer that surrounds the Blastocyst (early embryo) as it develops. Sperm must pass through the zona to fertilize the egg; once fertilization occurs, the zona reaction blocks all other sperm from entering (e.g., prevents polyspermy).

Zygote: A fertilized egg before any cell divisions have occurred. The first stage in the development of a baby. This is what the developing baby is called immediately after conception has occurred, while it is still in the fallopian tube of the mother.

BIBLIOGRAPHY

American Cancer Society: *http://www.cancer.org/*

Ariel, I. et al. (1994) "Relaxation of Imprinting in Trophoblastic Disease." *Gynecologic Oncology* 53: 212-219.

Armstrong, D. (2001) "Exploring Fathers' Experiences of Pregnancy After a Prior Perinatal Loss." *The American Journal of Maternal/Child Nursing* 26(3) May/June: 147-153.

BBC News (2002) "Cloned Baby Warning." Wednesday, 10 April, 2002 *http://news.bbc.co.uk/1/hi/health/1921205.stm* (retrieved 05/16/03)

Berkowitz, R. and D. P. Goldstein (1989) "Gestational Trophoblastic Diseases." *Seminars in Oncology* 16(5): 410-416, October.

Berkowitz, R. et al. (1984) "Choriocarcinoma following Term Gestation." *Gynecologic Oncology*, 17: 52-57.

Berkowitz, R. et al. (2000) "Management of Gestational Trophoblastic Disease: Subsequent Pregnancy Experience." *Seminars in Oncology* 27(6) December: 678-685.

Bourgeois Law, G. and R. Lotocki (1999) "Sexuality and Gynaecological Cancer: A Needs Assessment" *Canadian Journal Of Human Sexuality* 8(4): 231-240.

Bower, M. et al. (1995) "Gestational Choriocarcinoma." *Annals of Oncology* 6(5): 503-508.

Buckley, J. (1984) "The Epidemiology of Molar Pregnancy and Choriocarcinoma." *Clinical Obstetrics and Gynecology* 27(1) March.

Burstein, H. (2000) "Discussing Complementary Therapies With Cancer Patients: What Should We Be Talking About?" *Journal of Clinical Oncology* 18(13) July: 2501-2504.

Bygdeman, M. and K. Danielsson (2002) "Options for Early Therapeutic Abortion: A Comparative Review." *Drugs* 62(17): 2459-2470.

Canadian Association of Nurses in Oncology *Feeling Your Best: A self-help guide for cancer patients.* GlaxoSmithKline.

Canadian Cancer Society (1999) *Chemotherapy and You: A Guide to Self Help During Treatment.*

Canadian Cancer Society (2001) *Taking Time: Support for people living with cancer and people who care about them.*

Canadian Cancer Society (2001) *The Nutrition Guide for People Living with Cancer: A resource for people with cancer, their families and their friends.*

CancerBackup: *http://www.cancerbacup.org.uk/*

Cheung, A. et al. (1999) "Telomerase activity in gestational trophoblastic disease." *Journal of Clinical Pathology* 52(8) August: 588-592.

Cohn, D. and T. Herzog (2000) "Gestational trophoblastic diseases: new standards for therapy." *Current Opinion in Oncology* 12(5) September: 492-496.

Colls, B M. (2000) "Tumour markers in malignancies… as are monoclonal immunoglobulin and [beta] human chorionic gonadotrophin." *BMJ: The British Medical Journal* 321(7257) August 5th: 380.

Cote-Arsenault, D. and D. Bidlack (2001) "Women's Emotions and Concerns During Pregnancy Following Perinatal Loss." *The American Journal of Maternal/Child Nursing* 26(3) May/June: 128-134.

De Marquiegui, A. and M. Huish (1999) "ABC of Sexual Health: A Woman's Sexual Life After an Operation." *BMJ: British Medical Journal* 318(7177) January 16th: 178-181.

Deadman, J.M. et al.. (2001) "Taking Responsibility For Cancer Treatment" *Social Science and Medicine* 53(5) September: 669-677.

Dizon-Townson, D. et al. (2000) "Genetic Expression by Fetal Chorionic Villi During the First Trimester of Human Gestation." *American Journal of Obstetrics and Gynecology* 183(3) September: 706-711.

Dobson, L.S. et al. (2000) "Persistent Gestational Trophoblastic Disease: Results of MEA (methotrexate, etopiside and dactinomycin) as first-line chemotherapy in high risk disease and EA (etopiside and dactinomycin) as second-line therapy for low risk disease." *British Journal of Cancer* 82(9): 1547-1552.

Ferrell, Betty R. et al. (1995) "Quality of Life in Long-Term Cancer Survivors." *Oncology Nursing Forum* 22(6): 915-922.

Finkler, N. (1991) "Placental Site Trophoblastic Tumor: Diagnosis, Clinical Behaviour and Treatment." *The Journal of Reproductive Medicine* 36(1) January: 27-30.

Gillespie, A.M. et al. (2000) "Placental Site Trophoblastic Tumor: a rare but potentially curable cancer." *The British Journal of Cancer* 82(6): 1186-1190.

Gillespie, A. S. Kumar and B.W. Hancock. (2000) "Treatment of Persistenet Trophoblastic Disease Later Than 6 Months after Diagnosis of Molar Pregnancy." *British Journal of Cancer* 82(8): 1393-1395.

Hemsley Robinson, B. (1994) "Intraoperative Molar Pregnancy Crisis." *AORN Journal* 60(2) August: 193-201.

Hudson, T. (2002) "Perimenopause Naturally: An Integrative Medicine Approach." *A Friend Indeed* XVIII (6) January: 1.

Hughes, M. "Sexuality Issues: Keeping Your Cool." *Oncology Nursing Forum* 23(10): 1597-1600, 1996.

Hui, P. et al. (2000) "Pathogenesis of Placental Site Trophoblastic Tumor May Require the Presence of a Paternally Derived X Chromosome." *Laboratory Investigation* 80(6) June: 965-972.

Ino, K. et al. (2001) "Complete Remission of Gestational Choriocarcinoma with Choroidal Metastasis Treated with Systemic Chemotherapy Alone: Case Report and Review of Literature." *Gynecologic Oncology* 83: 601-604.

Irvine, D. et al. (1994) "The Prevalence and Correlates of Fatigue in Patients receiving Treatment with Chemotherapy and Radiotherapy: A comparison with the fatigue experienced by healthy individuals." *Cancer Nursing* 17(5): 367-378.

Jin, M. et al. (2001) "Expression of Serine Protinase Inhibitor PP5/TFPI-2/MSPI Decreases the Invasive Potential of Human Choriocarcinoma Cells in Vitro and in Vivo." *Gynecologic Oncology*, 83: 325-333.

Jones, H. W. III. (2002) "Placental Site Trophoblastic Tumor: A 17-Year Experience at the New England Trophoblastic Disease Center." *Obstetrical & Gynecological Survey* 57(1) January: 28-29.

Jones, et al. (1996) "Case Report: Treatment of Resistant Gestational Choriocarcinoma with Taxol: A Report of Two Cases." *Gynecologic Oncology* 61: 126-130.

Jonquil, S. (1996) "Molar Pregnancy: A Case Study and Review." *Midwifery Today* 35, Fall.

Josefson, D. (2001) "Infertility experts offer new hope to women having cancer treatment." *BMJ: The British Medical Journal* 323(7316) October 6th: 769.

Kaczan-Bourgois, D. J. Salles and H. Chap (1999) "Expression of annexin II and associated p11 protein by differentiated choriocarcinoma Jar cells." *American Journal of Obstetrics & Gynecology* 181(5) November: 1273.

Kale, A. et al. (2001) "Expression of Proliferation Markers (Ki-67, proliferating cell nuclear antigen, and silver-staining nucleolar organizer regions) and of p53 tumor Protein in Gestational Trophoblastic Disease." *American Journal of Obstetrics and Gynecology* 184(4) March: 567-574.

Kendall, A. R. Gillmore and E. Newlands (2002) "Chemotherapy for trophoblastic disease: current standards." *Current Opinion in Obstetrics & Gynecology* 14(1) February: 33-38.

Khastgir, G. and J. Studd (2000) "Patients' outlook, experience, and satisfaction with hysterectomy, bilateral oophorectomy, and subsequent continuation of hormone replacement therapy." *American Journal of Obstetrics & Gynecology* 183(6) December: 1427-1433.

Kohorn, E. (1995) "The Trophoblastic Tower of Babel: Classification Systems for Metastatic Gestational Trophoblastic Neoplasia." *Gynecologic Oncology* 56: 280-288.

Kohorn, Ernest I. (2000) "Measurement of CA-125 in Trophoblastic Disease." *Gynecologic Oncology*, 78: 39-42.

Kohorn, E. (2003) "The FIGO 2000 Staging and Risk Factor Scoring System for Gestational Trophoblastic Neoplasia." *Gestational Trophoblastic Disease, 2nd Edition.* B. W. Hancock, E. S. Newlands, R. S. Berkowitz and L. A. Cole (eds.) International Society for the Study of Trophoblastic Disease (ISSTD) *http://www.isstd.org/gtd/index.html* (accessed 09/15/05).

Kurtz, M. et al. (1995) "Relationship of Caregiver Reactions and Depression to Cancer Patients' Symptoms, Functional States and Depression - A Longitudinal View" *Social Science and Medicine* 40(6) March: 837-846.

Lan, Z. et al. (2001) "Pregnancy Outcomes of Patients Who Conceived within 1 Year after Chemotherapy for Gestational Trophoblastic Tumor: A Clinical Report of 22 Patients." *Gynecologic Oncology* 83: 146-148.

Li H.W. S.W. Tsao and A.N. Cheung. (2002) "Current Understandings of the Molecular Genetics of Gestational Trophoblastic Diseases." *Placenta* 23(1) January: 20-31.

Lorigan, P.C. et al. (2000) "Characteristics of Women with Recurrent Molar Pregnancies." *Gynecologic Oncology* 78: 288-292.

Love, P. and J. Robinson (1994) *Hot Monogamy: Essential Steps to More Passionate, Intimate Lovemaking.* A Plume Book: New York.

Lowdermilk, D. and B. Germino (2000) "Helping Women and Their Families Cope with the Impact of Gynecologic Cancer." *JOGNN: Journal of Obstetric, Gynecologic and Neonatal Nursing* 29(6) November/December: 653-660.

Mangili, G. et. al. (1996) "Management of Low-Risk Gestational Trophoblastic Tumors with Etopiside (VP16) in Patients Resistant to Methotrexate." *Gynecologic Oncology* 61: 218-220.

Markman, M. "Safety Issues in Using Complementary and Alternative Medicine." *Journal of Clinical Oncology.* 20(18s) SUPPLEMENT: 39s-41s, September 15, 2002.

Matsui, H. et al. (2000) "Combination Chemotherapy with Methotrexate, Etopiside, and Actinomycin D for High-Risk Gestational Trophoblastic Tumors." *Gynecologic Oncology* 78: 28-31.

National Cancer Institute, *http://www.nci.nih.gov/*

Newlands, E. S. et al. (2000) "Etoposide and Cisplatin/Etoposide, Methotrexate, and Actinomycin D (EMA) Chemotherapy for Patients with High-Risk Gestational Trophoblastic Tumors Refractory to EMA/Cyclophosphamide and Vincristine Chemotherapy and Patients Presenting with Metastatic Placental Site Trophoblastic Tumors." *Journal of Clinical Oncology* 18(4) February: 854-859.

Odunsi, K.O. (1998) "Necrosis of Myometrial Choriocarcinoma with Fulminating Sepsis Complicating Chemotherapy for Trophoblastic Tumor." *Gynecologic Oncology* 70: 100-104.

Oktay, K. et al. (2001) "Endocrine Function and Oocyte Retrieval After Autologous Transplantation of Ovarian Cortical Strips to the Forearm." *JAMA: Journal Of The American Medical Association* 286(12) September 26: 1490-1493.

O'Leary Cobb, J. (1993) "Premature Menopause" *A Friend Indeed* 8(9) February: 1.

Olsen, J. et al. (1999) "Molar Pregnancy and Risk for Cancer in Women and Their Male Partners." *American Journal of Obstetrics and Gynecology* 181(3) September: 630-634.

Paul, M. et al. (2002) "Early surgical abortion: Efficacy and safety." *American Journal of Obstetrics & Gynecology* 187(2) August: 407-411.

Peters, J. et al. (2001) "Cancer Genetics Fundamentals" *Cancer Nursing* 24(6) December: 446-461.

Rannestad, T. et al. (2001) "The Quality of Life in Women Suffering from Gynecological Disorders is Improved by Means of Hysterectomy: Absolute and Relative Differences Between Pre- and Postoperative Measures." *Acta Obstetricia et Gynecologica Scandinavica* 80(1) January: 46-51.

Rauch, P. et al. (2002) "Parents With Cancer: Who's Looking After the Children?" *Journal of Clinical Oncology* 20(21) November: 4399-4402.

Rhodes, J. et al.. (1999) "Hysterectomy and Sexual Functioning." *JAMA: Journal Of The American Medical Association* 282(20) November 24th: 1934-1941.

Rich, W. "Gestational Trophoblastic Disease" *CancerLink http://www.personal.u-net.com/~njh/cgest.html (retrieved 04/21/02)*

Ridley, M. (1999) Genome: *The Autobiography of a Species in 23 Chapters* HarperCollins: New York.

Riegert-Johnson, D. D. McClary and B. McIver (2001) "Gestational Trophoblastic Disease: Another Cause of Nausea and Vomiting in Pregnancy." *Mayo Clinic Proceedings* 76(5) May: 566.

Roberts, N (2000) "Induced Menopause" *A Friend Indeed* XVII(2) May: 1.

Rosenthal, M.S. (1997) "Chapter 9: Friends and Lovers" in *The Breast Sourcebook: Everything You Need to Know about Cancer Detection, Treatment and Prevention.* Lowell House: Los Angeles.

RxList: *http://www.rxlist.com/*

Salisbury, A. et al. (2003) "Maternal-Fetal Attachment." *JAMA: Journal of the American Medical Association* 289(13) April 2nd: 1701.

Schou, K. et al. (2001) "Experiencing Cancer: Quality of Life in Treatment" *Journal Of Health Politics, Policy And Law* 26(4) August: 789-794.

Schuler-Maloney, D. and S. Lee "Placental Triage." *http://showcase.netins.net/web/placenta/* (retrieved 02/22/02)

Soper, JT. et al. (2004) "Diagnosis and Treatment of Gestational Trophoblastic Disease: ACOG Practice Bulletin No. 53," *Gynecologic Oncology* 93: 575-585.

Soto-Wright, V. et al. (1997) "The Management of Gestational Trophoblastic Tumors with Etopiside, Methotrexate, and Actinomycin D." *Gynecologic Oncology* 64: 156-159.

Steensma, D. (2002) "Why Me?" *Journal of Clinical Oncology* 20(3) February 1st: 873-875.

Stirrat, G. "Hydatidiform Mole" in *The Miscarriage Association: Acknowledging Pregnancy Loss. http://www.miscarriageassociation.org.uk/leaflets/hydamole.pdf* (retrieved 05/16/03)

Szulman, A. (2000) "Choriocarcinoma after hydatidiform mole." *American Journal of Obstetrics & Gynecology* 183(1) July: 257.

Taniguchi, F. et al. (2000) "Keratinocyte growth factor in the promotion of human chorionic gonadotropin production in human choriocarcinoma cells." *American Journal of Obstetrics & Gynecology* 182(3) March: 692-698.

Thomas, C. S Morris and J. Harman (2002) "Companions Through Cancer: the care given by informal carers in cancer contexts" *Social Science and Medicine* 54(4) February: 529-544.

Tidy, J.A. et al. (2000) "Gestational Trophoblastic Disease: A Study of Mode of Evacuation and Subsequent Need for Treatment with Chemotherapy." *Gynecologic Oncology* 78: 309-312.

Trisdale, S.K. (2002) "Working with your Doctor" WORLD: 3, April.

Tuncer, Z. et al. (1999) "Outcome of Pregnancies Occurring Before Completion of Human Chorionic Gonadotropin Follow-Up in Patients with Persistent Gestational Trophoblastic Tumor." *Obstetrical & Gynecological Survey* 54(10) October: 639-640.

University of Newcastle upon Tyne: "On-Line Medical Dictionary" *http://cancerweb.ncl.ac.uk/omd/*

Von Gruenigen, V. E. et al. (2001) "A comparison of complementary and alternative medicine use by gynecology and gynecologic oncology patients." *International Journal of Gynecological Cancer* 11(3) May/June: 205-209.

Wade, J. et al. (2000) "Hysterectomy: What Do Women Need and Want to Know?" *JOGNN - Journal of Obstetric, Gynecologic, & Neonatal Nursing* 29(1) January/February: 33-42.

Walsgrove, H (2001) "Hysterectomy." *Nursing Standard* 15(29) April 4th: 47-55.

Wang, P.H. et al. (1997) "The VIP Regimen Effective Treatment to Refractory Choriocarcinoma: A Case Report" *Chinese Medical Journal (Taipei)* 59: 320-4. *http://www.vghtpe.gov.tw/~cmj/5905/590509.htm* (retrieved 10/16/02)

Wang, Y. et al. (1998) "Chemotherapy Using 5-Fluorouracil and Nitrocaphanum in Malignant Trophoblastic Tumor" *Gynecologic Oncology* 71: 416-419.

Wilber, K. (1988) "On Being A Support Person." *The Journal of Transpersonal Psychology* 20(2): 141-159.

Wilmoth, M.C. and A. Spinelli (2000) "Sexual Implications of Gynecologic Cancer Treatments." *JOGNN: Journal of Obstetric, Gynecologic and Neonatal Nursing* 29(4) July/August: 413-421.

Wong, L.C. et al. (2000) "Methotrexate Infusion in Low-Risk Gestational Trophoblastic Disease." *American Journal of Obstetrics & Gynecology* 183(6) December: 1579-1582.

Wongweragiat, S. R. Searle and J. Bulmer (1999) "Decidual T Lymphocyte Activation in Hydatidiform Mole." *Journal of Clinical Pathology* 52(12) December: 888-894.

Woolas, R. et al. (1999) "Influence of Chemotherapy for Gestational Trophoblastic Disease on Subsequent Pregnancy Outcome." *Obstetrical & Gynecological Survey* 54(2) February: 108-109.

INDEX

Miscarriage, 12, 16, 18, 28, 31, 46, 95, 211, 214

Molar pregnancy, 16, 19, 26, 28–31, 33–35, 48, 52, 85, 209–210

Mole,

Complete, 26–27, 44, 50, 209

Invasive, 19, 26, 30, 34, 86, 217, 220

Metastatic, 19, 26, 30, 87

Partial, 26, 28–29, 50, 209

Persistent, 26, 30, 86

Muscle, 32, 123, 145, 157, 166, 222, 224–225

N

Nausea, 51, 122–127, 143, 151, 160, 216

Nerve, 54, 56, 144, 161

Neupogen, 70, 88, 104, 113, 169

Nurse, 14, 47, 57, 62, 65, 104–105, 114, 117, 123, 126, 131, 148, 155

Nutrition, 14–15, 47, 57, 62, 65, 104–105, 114–115, 117, 123, 126, 131, 148, 155

O

Obstetrician-Gynecologist (OBGYN), 12–13, 63, 75, 93, 223

Oncogenes, 38, 41, 43–44, 223

Ovaries, 14, 27, 50, 85, 95–97, 100, 143, 199, 220, 222–223

P

Pain, 50, 56, 59, 119–120, 218

Pap smear, 63, 96

Pelvic exam, 61–63

Peripherally inserted central catheter

(PICC Line), 106

Persistent GTN, 30, 34

Placenta, 12–13, 19–26, 31–32, 34, 43–44, 50, 61, 83, 92, 192, 210, 224–226

Placental site trophoblastic tumor (PSTT), 26, 32

Platelets, 70, 75, 112, 115–116, 216

Port, 105–106

Pregnancy,

Abnormal, 26–35, 73–74, 218

After GTN treatment, 209–211

Emotions and loss, 93–95, 163

Full-term or normal, 16, 24, 44, 51–52, 60, 68, 82, 91, 202, 220

Molar, 16, 19, 26, 28–31, 33–35, 48, 50, 52, 85, 90, 209–210, 222

R

Recurrence, 18, 38, 81, 202, 208–209

Recurrent GTN, 92, 210

Relationship, 26, 75, 94, 110, 160, 164, 167, 177, 179, 199, 209

Remission, 16, 32, 38, 84, 86, 88, 90, 92, 102, 201–203, 208–209

S

Secondary cancer, 203

Sex, 50, 82, 91, 98–100, 142–143, 163–167, 172, 220

Side effect, 117, 119, 122, 132, 134, 139–140, 149–151, 218

Staging system, 60, 70–72, 80, 90

Stress, 16, 18, 94, 107, 144, 147, 153, 156–158, 161, 167, 170, 188, 206, 208

Support,
> Children and, 179, 184
> Emotional, 107, 211
> Fathers/partners and, 95, 167, 170–175, 214
> Family, friends and, 186, 188, 195, 197
> Group, 18, 46, 152–153, 155, 172–174, 204, 214
> and Miscarriage, 94, 211, 214

Surgery,
> Personal experience, 14, 106, 159, 176, 187, 192–193
> Use in treatment, 28, 29, 83–89, 91, 92–101
> *see also* Hysterectomy, Dilation and curettage (D&C)

Survivor, 18, 36, 211–212

T

Taxol, 83, 112, 118
Trophoblast, 22–23, 218, 221, 225–226
Tumor, 14, 32, 37–38, 41–45, 48, 50, 53–54, 58, 71–74, 92–93, 102, 104–105, 149, 216, 218, 220, 222,–224
Tumor suppressor genes, 38, 41–42, 44

U

Ultrasound, 12, 14, 32, 49, 66, 72–73, 95, 175, 210, 219
Urinary tract, 145–146
Urine, 52, 58–59, 69, 145–146, 224
Uterine wall, 14, 29–30, 48, 92

Uterus, 14, 21–23, 25, 29–32, 34, 50–52, 54, 56, 58–59, 62, 72, 80, 85–86, 92–93, 95–98, 104–105, 141, 162, 199, 216, 218, 220–224, 226

V

Vagina, 48, 50, 57–58, 62–63, 66, 72, 97–98, 100, 115, 142, 163, 166–167, 220, 226
Vaginal dryness, 116, 142, 165
Vincristine, 88, 90, 149
Vitamins, 102, 110, 159
Vomiting, 14, 48, 51–53, 104, 118, 122–126, 151, 216

W

Weight loss, 55
Womb, 95, 98, 200, 222, 226

X

X-ray, 64, 72–73, 162, 217, 221

Z

Zygote, 20–21

Made in the USA
Columbia, SC
22 January 2021

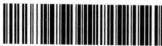

31404483R00133